Practical Echocardiography
for Cardiac Sonographers

NOTICE

Medicine is an ever-changing science. As new research and clinical experience broaden our knowledge, changes in treatment and drug therapy are required. The authors and the publisher of this work have checked with sources believed to be reliable in their efforts to provide information that is complete and generally in accord with the standards accepted at the time of publication. However, in view of the possibility of human error or changes in medical sciences, neither the authors nor the publisher nor any other party who has been involved in the preparation or publication of this work warrants that the information contained herein is in every respect accurate or complete, and they disclaim all responsibility for any errors or omissions or for the results obtained from use of the information contained in this work. Readers are encouraged to confirm the information contained herein with other sources. For example and in particular, readers are advised to check the product information sheet included in the package of each drug they plan to administer to be certain that the information contained in this work is accurate and that changes have not been made in the recommended dose or in the contraindications for administration. This recommendation is of particular importance in connection with new or infrequently used drugs.

Practical Echocardiography for Cardiac Sonographers

Daniel M. Shindler, MD, FACC
Professor of Medicine
Rutgers Robert Wood Johnson Medical School
New Brunswick, New Jersey

Olga I. Shindler, MD
President, Mobile Cardiac Ultrasound Inc.
East Brunswick, New Jersey
Editor, Hand-Held Echocardiography Journal
Efslope.com

Alicia Wright, RCS
Clinical Instructor, Cardiac Sonography Program
Rutgers School of Health Professions
Clinical Lead Sonographer, Echocardiography Laboratory
Robert Wood Johnson University Hospital
New Brunswick, New Jersey

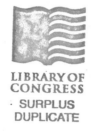

New York   Chicago   San Francisco   Lisbon   London   Madrid   Mexico City   New Delhi
San Juan   Seoul   Singapore   Sydney   Toronto

PRACTICAL ECHOCARDIOGRAPHY FOR CARDIAC SONOGRAPHERS

1 2 3 4 5 6 7 8 9   LCR   25 24 23 22 21 20

ISBN 978-1-260-45779-7
MHID 1-260-45779-6

This book was set in Minion Pro by Aptara, Inc.

The editors were Karen Edmonson and Christie Naglieri.

The production supervisor was Catherine Saggese.

Project management was provided by Dinesh Pokhriyal.

This book is printed on acid-free paper.

Library of Congress Cataloging-in-Publication Data

Library of Congress Control Number: 2019951838

Cataloging in Publication data available on request from publisher.

McGraw Hill books are available at special quantity discounts to use as premiums and sales promotions, or for use in corporate training programs. To contact a representative please visit the Contact Us pages at www.mhprofessional.com.

Daniel and Olga Shindler dedicate this book to the countless sonographers who have challenged and inspired us with their insightful questions for over three decades.

Alicia Wright would like to extend love and gratitude to her husband Stan, two daughters Tya'Seanah and Tyara, and to her mother Emma McRae for their constant support, and for always being there when she needs them.

Contents

Videos are located at **mhprofessional.com/practicalecho**

Introduction

This is a practical reference that serves to introduce the discipline of echocardiography. It is meant to be integrated with the search capabilities of a modern cell phone. It enables the reader to quickly find, understand, and quote the relevant literature.

The book stems from more than 30 busy years in an academic echocardiography laboratory, and from our initial efforts starting in 1994 to provide free echocardiography education and to promote social media discussions of echocardiography on the Internet.

Topics are succinctly presented to introduce basic concepts and proper terminology. They stem from the ongoing monthly sonographer education meetings of the Central Jersey Echo Society that started in 1989.

Relevant references were carefully selected and added where appropriate. They are meant to introduce the reader to the vast literature of echocardiography. They are provided to serve as a source of further reading. Many are annotated or have keywords in bold. Some references are historic and show the evidence-based foundations of echocardiography.

Most references are easily accessible by using the search capabilities of a smartphone. They can also be easily copied and pasted into the Google Scholar search box.

The best way to learn echocardiography is to see multiple versions and variations of important echo findings. Echo clips in this book can be accessed by reading QR codes with a cell phone camera app, or by using a Web browser.

Existing echocardiography guidelines are not duplicated in this book. Instead, guideline documents are referenced and annotated. Guideline apps should be downloaded by the reader and kept close at hand. Once downloaded, the best way to start with an echo guideline document is to review the images. The videos in this book were chosen to supplement guideline images. Transesophageal videos can be recognized by the angle icon at the top of the screen.

The authors wish to thank Karen Edmonson from McGraw Hill for the constant encouragement and support.

Daniel M. Shindler, MD, FACC
Olga I. Shindler, MD
Alicia Wright, RCS

CHAPTER 1

Ultrasound

DEFINITION OF ULTRASOUND

- Sound *frequencies* above the audible range.
- Familiar example: A dog whistle.

TRANSDUCER FREQUENCY (PITCH)

- Units: MHz—million (mega) cycles (Hz) per second.
- Examples of typical clinical transducers:
  - Low-frequency transducers are physically bigger ("woofers") and emit around 2 MHz.
  - High-frequency transducers are physically smaller ("tweeters") and emit around 5 or 7.5 MHz.
- Frequency is picked by manually choosing the transducer and/or by setting the frequency electronically in the chosen transducer.
- The frequency choice affects image quality:
  - Lower frequency penetrates deeper, but the images are more "coarse."
  - Higher frequency provides better resolution but less penetration.
  - The settings of modern multifrequency transducers are electronically altered by the user for desired results: deeper penetration versus better resolution.

ULTRASOUND TRANSDUCERS

- Ultrasound transducers are used for echocardiographic imaging. Electricity is converted to ultrasound by a transducer and *transmitted* to the body.
- *Reflected* sound from cardiac tissue is converted back to electrical signals by the same transducer. The reflected signals are used to create a visual display of cardiac anatomy, and to perform Doppler calculations of cardiac physiology.
- Familiar transducer back-and-forth example using *audible* sound:
  - Sound is converted to electricity by a microphone.
  - Electricity is converted back to sound by sending it to a speaker.

- Ultrasound transducers use the piezoelectric effect: A ceramic material vibrates and produces ultrasound waves when an electrical current is passed through it.

TRANSDUCER MANIPULATION

- There are five basic transducer movements:
  - Sliding, rocking, tilting, rotation, and compression.
  - Transducer motion that is perpendicular to the visualized plane is called *cross-plane motion.*
  - Rotating the transducer from 11 o'clock to 2 o'clock switches from long to short axis.

American Institute of Ultrasound in Medicine. Transducer manipulation for echocardiography. J Ultrasound Med. 2005; 24:733–736.

PHYSICAL PROPERTIES OF ULTRASOUND

- Sound is a mechanical wave.
- In order for sound to propagate, it must travel through a medium.
- Sound *starts* with a vibrating object that pushes and pulls adjacent molecules.
- Sound *spreads* by propagating these vibrations to still farther molecules.
- The movie *Alien* was promoted with the slogan "In space no one can hear you scream." As opposed to light, sound cannot travel through the vacuum of outer space.
- The direction of sound waves is longitudinal. In other words, sound makes the medium vibrate back and forth in the direction that it travels. Think of the visible to-and-fro movements made by the membrane of a large sound speaker, and how it compresses and decompresses the air in front of it.
- Sound propagation results in regions of compression and regions of rarefaction (decompression) within the medium through which the sound is traveling.
- When sound travels through tissues, there can be mechanical and thermal effects on the tissue.

CAVITATION

"Formation of gas bubbles in blood during the rarefaction phase."

SCANNING TIPS FOR CAVITATION

- Cavitation can be found in patients with mechanical mitral or prosthetic aortic valves.
- In these cases, cavitation is typically best demonstrated when harmonic imaging is turned on.

MECHANICAL INDEX

- The mechanical index indicates the amount of sound energy delivered during tissue *rarefaction* (expansion after being compressed by the sound energy).

- The mechanical index is adjustable on ultrasound machines.
- It needs to be adjusted *downward* during imaging of contrast bubbles to avoid bubble destruction.
- Changing transducer frequency affects the mechanical index.
  - It is an inverse relationship.
  - The lower the frequency, the higher the mechanical index.
- True echocardiographers think of the mechanical index every time they open a bottle of soda after shaking it.

Porter TR, Xie F, Silver M, et al. Real-time **perfusion imaging** with low mechanical index pulse inversion Doppler imaging. J Am Coll Cardiol. 2001;37:748–753.

WAVELENGTH

- Wavelength is important to understand when thinking about the travel of ultrasound through tissue.
- Wavelength is a *distance* between regions of compression and regions of rarefaction in tissue.
- It is the distance of one ultrasound cycle.
- Wavelength should not be confused with period.
- Wavelength is written with units of *distance*: cm, mm, etc.
- Period is written with units of *time*: seconds, milliseconds, etc.
- Tip: Remember the phrase *period of time*.
- The relationship of wavelength and frequency:
  - **Frequency** is cycles per unit of time.
  - **Wavelength** is the distance of one cycle.
  - **Period** is the time spent to complete one cycle.
- Image resolution tips:
  - The importance of wavelength is the relationship to image resolution.
  - A short wavelength provides better image resolution.
  - Wavelength is determined by tissue density and by ultrasound frequency.
  - The operator cannot change the density of tissue being examined.
  - Hence, when frequency is being changed by the user, this is also the only way to affect the wavelength.
- The relationship between wavelength and frequency is reciprocal:
  - Increasing frequency decreases wavelength and improves resolution.
  - Decreasing frequency increases wavelength and degrades resolution.
- Decreasing the frequency is often necessary to improve tissue penetration.

IMAGING TIP

- Changing the transducer frequency while watching the ultrasound image is extremely effective and should be done constantly during a study.

PERIOD

- Pulse repetition period *changes* during the echocardiographic examination.
- The shorter the distance from the transducer, the shorter the period (less time spent traveling from and back to the transducer).

AMPLITUDE, POWER, AND INTENSITY

- Electrical voltage is an example of a measure of **amplitude**.
- When a given voltage amplitude is applied to the ultrasound transducer, a proportionate amount of ultrasound power is applied to the body.
- **Power** is a measure of work carried out by the transducer. The units are the familiar Watts, the same as in a light bulb.
- The concentration of the power per square area is called the **intensity**.
- Familiar example of the importance of intensity:
  - A measured amount of rainfall can be loosely compared to power.
  - Amount of rain *per square area* is more comparable to intensity.
  - Importance of intensity: A hurricane may destroy a small area of land compared with the total amount of rainfall delivered by the hurricane.
- Intensity is important when thinking about bioeffects and ultrasound safety.

HARMONIC IMAGING

"Ultrasound returning from tissue contains new, higher-pitch ultrasound vibrations that are a multiple of the original transmitting frequency."

- As ultrasound travels through tissue, the mechanical energy of the transmitted ultrasound vibrations also creates *new* higher-frequency vibrations called harmonics.
- A familiar example of an audible sound and its harmonics is the complex and pleasant sound generated by a piano note.
- Harmonics are multiples of the original transducer frequency. Thus, the energy of a 2.5-MHz transducer will cause tissue to vibrate and emit 5-MHz, 10-MHz, and 20-MHz harmonic ultrasound signals that travel back to the transducer.
- The 2× multiple of the original frequency is the *first* harmonic.
- This tissue-created first harmonic only travels one way through the body: back to the transducer (not back and forth).
- The one-way travel provides less opportunity to scatter the ultrasound and create artifacts in comparison with a round trip.
- Harmonic imaging is used to reduce the amount of ultrasound artifacts, and to improve image quality.
- With the touch of a button on the ultrasound machine, it is possible to display only the returning first harmonic: harmonic imaging.
- The original lower frequency, called the *fundamental* frequency, is filtered out, and the echocardiographic image is created from the first harmonic.
- Familiar example of one-way *light wave* travel improving image resolution:

If you turn on the porch light, you can see the outside better through a screen door than if you turn on the indoor lights. The screen gets to scatter the light only one way from the outside back to your eye.

- Another way to understand the benefit of harmonic imaging is as follows:
  - Strong fundamental signals produce strong harmonics, whereas weak fundamental signals produce *very* weak harmonic signals. The weak fundamental signals are usually the undesirable scattered, artifact-producing signals, and their even weaker harmonics are less likely to create image artifacts.
  - Furthermore, harmonics are strongest at just the right distances used by imaging, and weakest near the transducer where more artifacts are generated. Hence, harmonic imaging has *fewer* near-field artifacts than fundamental imaging.

Anvari A, Forsberg F, Samir AE. A primer on the physical principles of tissue harmonic imaging. Radiographics. 2015;35:1955–1964.

Thomas JD, Rubin DN. Tissue harmonic imaging: why does it work? J Am Soc Echocardiogr. 1998;11:803–808.

Echoes most likely to produce artifacts are least likely to produce harmonic waves.

LOW-MECHANICAL-INDEX IMAGING

- There are different harmonic tissue cancellation techniques with different electronic approaches to overcome artifacts. They vary by ultrasound manufacturer and are important to understand when using ultrasound contrast agents with different brands of ultrasound equipment.
- Power modulation varies the ultrasound *amplitudes.*
- Pulse inversion sends pulses of alternating *polarity.*
- This is explained in detail in the guidelines below.

Porter TR, Mulvagh SL, Abdelmoneim SS, et al. Clinical applications of ultrasonic enhancing agents in echocardiography: 2018 American Society of Echocardiography Guidelines Update. J Am Soc Echocardiogr. 2018;31:241–274.

GRATING LOBES AND HARMONICS

- There are fewer grating lobe image artifacts with harmonics turned on.
- These artifacts are reflections due to weak, off-axis, undesirable ultrasound beams emitted by the transducer.
- Harmonic imaging results in weak reflections from the artifacts, and clear strong reflections from real anatomic structures.
- Some differences between grating lobe artifacts and side lobe artifacts:
  - Grating lobe artifacts are *ghost images* that are situated away from the main beam path. The artifactual image is placed at a wrong location.
  - Side lobe artifacts are located alongside the main ultrasound beam. They may be traceable to *small high-contrast reflectors* such as tissue or leaflet calcifications. These reflectors are often right in the path of the main ultrasound beam. The artifactual linear image is a sideways extension of the reflector. The origin

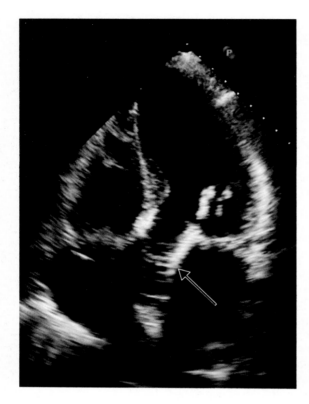

FIGURE 1-1. Artifacts from a TAVR prosthesis.

of the artifactual line can be visibly connected to the position of the anatomic reflector. An artifactual "line" created by a side lobe artifact may not be straight. It often has a subtle arc-like curve (Fig. 1-1).

- The proximal ascending aorta is notorious for sidelobe artifacts in the parasternal long axis (PLAX) view. They often create concerns about a possible dissection flap.
- Scanning tip: Turn harmonics on and off. Change the focus. Switch transducer frequencies.

*Buttery B, Davison G. The **ghost** artifact. J Ultrasound Med. 1984;3:49–52.*

*Ponnle A, Hasegawa H, Kanai H. Suppression of **grating lobe** artifacts in ultrasound images formed from diverging transmitting beams by modulation of receiving beams. Ultrasound Med Biol. 2013;39:681–691.*

*Rubin DN, Yazbek N, Garcia MJ, et al. Qualitative and quantitative effects of **harmonic** echocardiographic imaging on endocardial edge definition and **side-lobe** artifacts. J Am Soc Echocardiogr. 2000;13:1012–1018.*

COMPRESSION/DYNAMIC RANGE

- This is an important manual adjustment of the 2D echo image grayscale.
- It changes the relationship between the highest and lowest brightness levels in the echo image.

- The purpose is to fit many decibels of available ultrasound signals into the narrower visual range of the human eye.
- The grayscale bar on the side of the screen can show up to 256 shades of gray. The Compress button "fine tunes" how these 256 available shades of gray on the screen display the spectrum (dynamic range) of reflected ultrasound information.
- A high-compression, low-dynamic-range setting results in a high-contrast image that is mostly black and white with fewer grays in between. This is useful in difficult studies, to make the images less hazy and remove noise. Note: The membrane of the fossa ovalis in the apical four-chamber view may disappear.
- A low-compression, high-dynamic-range setting creates an image with more shades of gray. A smaller range of brightness levels is assigned to a particular shade of gray—hypothetically increasing the range, or spectrum of the anatomic information, but potentially also increasing image blurriness and noise. A "hazy, less contrasty" uniformly gray image may show important weaker signals such as valvular vegetations.
- Starting point: The default setting should have sufficient shades of gray to distinguish the transition between compacted and noncompacted myocardium.
- This setting should be constantly adjusted during a study. As stated above, it may make the difference between finding and missing a vegetation on a valve.
- It is important to know the expected difference between reducing *overall gain*, and reducing *dynamic range*:
  - Turning down overall gain is expected to reduce all ultrasound signals *equally*.
  - Turning down dynamic range should *preferentially* reduce clutter/noise signals with less effect on anatomic information.
- Explanation: Turning down the dynamic range can eliminate or reduce distinctly different low-level noise signals from scattered ultrasound reflections, while having little or no effect on higher level signals from true anatomic reflections.

Hangiandreou NJ. AAPM/RSNA **physics tutorial** for residents. Basic concepts and new technology. Radiographics. 2003; 23:1019–1033.

ULTRASOUND FORMULAS AND EQUATIONS

- Speed of sound in tissue = 1540 m/s = 0.154 cm/μs.
- The time to travel 2 cm = 2 ÷ 0.154 = 13 μs.
- Round-trip time to travel 1 cm back and forth in tissue = 13 μs.
- Time = Distance:
  - Ultrasound reflections are displayed at a certain *distance* from the transducer based on the *time* formulas above.
  - Wavelength = speed of sound (1540 m/s) ÷ frequency.
  - Wavelength and frequency are inversely related. The higher the one, the smaller the other.
  - The shorter the wavelength, the better the resolution.
  - The higher the frequency, the better the resolution.

- Nyquist limit of maximum measurable frequency = sample frequency ÷ 2.
- Doppler Formula:
  - The Doppler frequency shift is used to determine speed and direction of blood cells or moving myocardial tissue.
- However, it also depends on:
  - Transmitted frequency of ultrasound.
  - Speed of sound through tissue (1540 m/s).
  - Intercept angle between the transducer beam and the moving structure.
- Frequency: *Number* of ultrasound cycles in a given amount of time.
- Period: *Time* (duration) of one ultrasound cycle.
- Period = 1 ÷ frequency.
- Frequency = 1 ÷ period.
- Pulse repetition period = time from start of one pulse to the start of the next pulse (includes transmit time and listen time).
- Pulse repetition period = 13 μs × imaging distance in cm.
- Pulse repetition period = 1 ÷ pulse repetition frequency.
- Pulse repetition frequency = number of pulses transmitted into the body.
- Pulse repetition frequency = 1 ÷ pulse repetition period.
- Pulse duration = period × number of cycles in a pulse.
- Duty factor = pulse duration ÷ pulse repetition period.
  - The units of time cancel each other out.
  - Duty factor is reported as %.
  - Continuous wave Doppler has a duty factor of 100%.
  - Otherwise, duty factor is small. Ultrasound transducers spend most of their time listening, not transmitting.
- Power is proportional to the amplitude squared.
- A small increase in transducer voltage amplitude results in a large increase in ultrasound power output.
- Intensity = power ÷ cross-section of beam area.
- A small increase in transducer voltage amplitude results in a large increase in intensity.
- Lateral resolution = beam width.
- Beam width at the focal point = half the ultrasound crystal diameter.
- Longitudinal resolution = axial = depth = radial = range = front-to-back resolution.
- Spatial pulse length = wavelength × cycle number.
- Longitudinal resolution = spatial pulse length ÷ 2.

ULTRASOUND SAFETY

- Ultrasound is sound energy that is transmitted into the body.
- Heat is generated when ultrasound energy is absorbed (Fig. 1-2).

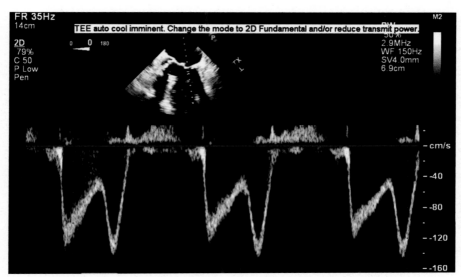

FIGURE 1-2. TEE probes left in a stationary position during open heart surgery may over-heat. Commercial ultrasound devices monitor this and generate shutdown warnings to prevent thermal damage to the esophagus.

- Heat produced depends on:
  - Duration of exposure. (Exposure with pulsed-wave Doppler is shorter than with continuous-wave Doppler.)
  - Tissue absorption of heat. (Blood flow in tissue can act as a coolant. Familiar example of variable absorption of light energy: Black absorbs more light than white.)
  - Acoustic energy (power and intensity).
- Acoustic power: Amount of acoustic energy per unit of time (like Watts in a light bulb).
- Intensity (power concentration): Acoustic power per unit of area (like high-intensity lamps that concentrate light): Watts/cm^2.
- Power divided by transducer surface area is used to compare quality of ultrasound devices.

The American Institute of Ultrasound in Medicine (AIUM.org) publishes a practical book on ultrasound safety.

Carstensen EL, Duck FA, Meltzer RS, et al. **Bioeffects** in echocardiography. Echocardiography. 1992;9:605–623.

O'Brien WD Jr. Ultrasound-biophysics mechanisms. Prog Biophys Mol Biol. 2007;93:212–255.

Mathematical overview.

Shankar H, Pagel PS. Potential adverse ultrasound-related **biological effects**: a critical review. Anesthesiology. 2011;115:1109–1124.

Skorton DJ, Collins SM, Greenleaf JF, et al. Ultrasound **bioeffects** and regulatory issues: an introduction for the echocardiographer. J Am Soc Echocardiogr. 1988;1:240–251.

ERGONOMICS

- Musculoskeletal disorders are a serious hazard to the health and safety of sonographers.
- Recommendations have been made on ways to reduce and prevent the frequency and severity of these disorders.
- Ultrasound societies are a good starting point for learning about injury prevention.

Horkey J, King P. Ergonomic **recommendations** and their role in cardiac sonography. Work. 2004;22:207–218.

Industry standards for the **prevention** of work-related musculoskeletal disorders in sonography. J Diagn Med Sonogr. 2017;33:370–391.

Mercer RB, Marcella CP, Carney DK, et al. Occupational health hazards to the ultrasonographer and their possible **prevention**. J Am Soc Echocardiogr. 1997;10:363–366.

Muir M, Hrynkow P, Chase R, et al. The nature, cause, and extent of occupational musculoskeletal injuries among sonographers: recommendations for **treatment** and prevention. J Diagn Med Sonogr. 2004;20:317–395.

Murphey S. Work related musculoskeletal disorders in sonography. J Diagn Med Sonogr. 2017;33:354–369.

Search **sdms.org** for ergonomics and Work-Related Musculoskeletal Disorders (**WRMSDs**) documents by this author.

Pike I, Russo A, Berkowitz J, et al. The **prevalence** of musculoskeletal disorders among diagnostic medical sonographers. J Diagn Med Sonogr. 1997;13:219–227.

Vanderpool HE, Friis EA, Smith BS, et al. Prevalence of **carpal tunnel** syndrome and other work-related musculoskeletal problems in cardiac sonographers. J Occup Med. 1993;35:604–610.

TWO-DIMENSIONAL IMAGING

- Anatomy is displayed as an echocardiographic image created *by multiple parallel ultrasound beams*. Multiple sound reflections are combined for this purpose.
- Historic note:
  - The first mode of ultrasound was A-mode (amplitude displayed as a series of lines).
  - This was followed by B-mode (amplitude displayed as brightness on an oscilloscope).
  - Then came M-mode (brightness displayed on moving paper).
  - Multiple M-mode beams were then combined to display a 2D anatomic slice.
  - A solid pyramid of 2D slices was subsequently combined for 3D imaging.

Cerqueira MD, Weissman NJ, Dilsizian V, et al. Standardized **myocardial segmentation** and nomenclature for tomographic imaging of the heart. Circulation. 2002;105:539–542.

Gardin JM, Adams DB, Douglas PS, et al. Recommendations for a **standardized report** for adult transthoracic echocardiography. J Am Soc Echocardiogr. 2002;15:275–290.

Hahn RT, Abraham T, Adams MS, et al. Guidelines for performing a comprehensive **transesophageal** echocardiographic examination. Anesth Analg. 2014;118:21–68.

Henry WL, DeMaria A, Gramiak R, et al. Report of the American Society of Echocardiography Committee on **nomenclature and standards** in two-dimensional echocardiography. Circulation. 1980;62:212–217.

Wharton G, Steeds R, Allen J, et al. A minimum dataset for a standard adult transthoracic echocardiogram: a **guideline protocol** from the British Society of Echocardiography. Echo Res Pract. 2015;2:G9–G24.

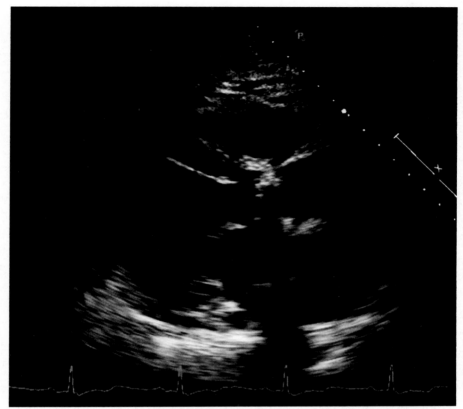

FIGURE 1-3. Reverberation, duplication, and attenuation created by an aortic prosthesis.

BEHAVIOR OF ULTRASOUND TRAVELING THROUGH TISSUE

Baad M, Lu ZF, Reiser I, et al. Clinical significance of US **artifacts**. Radiographics. 2017;37:1408–1423.

Excellent illustrations (Fig. 1-3).

Bertrand PB, Levine RA, Isselbacher EM, et al. Fact or **artifact** in two-dimensional echocardiography: avoiding misdiagnosis and missed diagnosis. J Am Soc Echocardiogr. 2016;29:381–391.

Le HT, Hangiandreou N, Timmerman R, et al. Imaging **artifacts** in echocardiography. Anesth Analg. 2016;122:633–646.

Prabhu SJ, Kanal K, Bhargava P, et al. Ultrasound **artifacts**: classification, applied physics with illustrations, and imaging appearances. Ultrasound Q. 2014;30:145–157.

Quien MM, Saric M. Ultrasound imaging **artifacts**: how to recognize them and how to avoid them. Echocardiography. 2018;35:1388–1401.

ATTENUATION ("Muffling")

- As ultrasound travels through tissue, the amplitude (sound energy strength) decreases.
- There is a greater decrease in amplitude with higher frequencies.

Units of Attenuation: Decibels

- Decibels are logarithmic (like the familiar Richter scale for earthquakes).
- Logarithms are used for *large changes in numbers* because of the large drop in ultrasound amplitude as it travels through the body.
- Even a small change in decibels still means a large change in ultrasound amplitude. A Richter 2 earthquake is barely perceptible. A Richter 8 earthquake destroyed San Francisco.
- Practical point: Because of the large logarithmic drop in signal amplitude, the user can amplify the weak deep distant ultrasound reflections with the time gain compensation (TGC) sliders that are present on ultrasound machines.

REFLECTION

- A portion of the transmitted ultrasound gets reflected back toward the transducer at boundaries of tissues with different densities.
- *Specular* reflection—the tissue acts as a "mirror" to ultrasound (Fig. 1-4).
- Example: The pericardium can behave like a specular reflector.
- In the parasternal long and short axis views, the pericardial reflection is typically the brightest component of the echocardiographic image.

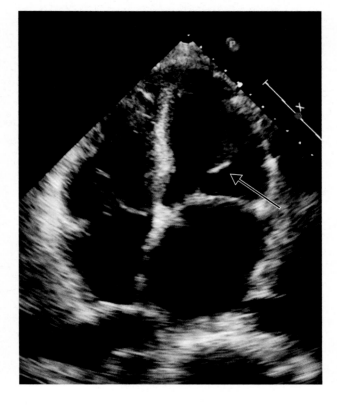

FIGURE 1-4. Specular reflection from a calcified papillary muscle tip.

- Reflection can create an extreme form of *attenuation*. Thus, in the example above, the pericardium in the parasternal long-axis view can sometimes reflect almost all of the ultrasound energy. This is similar to a mirror not allowing light waves to continue to travel past the mirror surface.
- As a result, in our example, no ultrasound reflections can come back to the transducer from tissues located past this portion of the pericardium. In such cases, there is no further anatomic information coming back to the transducer from tissue deeper than the pericardium. Everything in the ultrasound images located past the pericardium in these all-too-common cases is just an ultrasound artifact.

Adams MS, Alston TA. Echocardiographic reflections on a pericardium. Anesth Analg. 2007;104:506.

Perhaps because of calcification resulting from pericarditis, the pericardium of a patient was especially reflective and so permitted **unusual mirror images** *to be viewed. A pulsatile round mass was probably a mirror image of parts of the right ventricle. Sound beams reflected from the pericardium were carried up to the right ventricle. Echoes from right ventricular tissues were carried back to the transducer via another bounce on the pericardium.*

Because the pericardium functioned as a mirror, the artifactual image was displayed as if it existed beyond the pericardial reflector.

- A second descending aorta may get displayed during suprasternal imaging. An inferior vena cava may become duplicated in a subcostal view.

Adams MS, Alston TA. A **duplicate** inferior vena cava? J Cardiothorac Vasc Anesth. 2006;20:284–285.

- An example of the mechanism of a common upside-down **mirror image** artifact is as follows:
  - In the parasternal long axis view, a small amount of ultrasound manages to *continue past* the highly reflective posterior pericardium.
  - It subsequently reflects off a deeper structure and starts to return, striking the "back side" pleural surface of the posterior pericardium. The ultrasound then bounces back and forth at least one more time.
  - The ultrasound reflections that eventually make it back to the transducer are delayed. Time is distance, so they are displayed behind the heart.
  - The anatomy is upside down because of the "ping pong" process in step 2. It is displayed behind, and not on top of, the heart as explained in step 3.

Bertrand PB, Verhaert D, Vandervoort PM. Mirror artifacts in two-dimensional echocardiography: don't forget objects in the third dimension. J Am Soc Echocardiogr. 2015;28:1376–1377.

- Practical points for avoiding and understanding mirror artifacts:
  - Doppler and 2D imaging are at opposite ends for angle of incidence and information quality.
  - The best 2D images are obtained when ultrasound strikes tissue at 90 degrees (*perpendicular*).
  - The most accurate Doppler measurements are obtained when the measured movement of blood or tissue is at 0 degrees (*parallel*) to the ultrasound beam.

REFRACTION

- Like a light beam bouncing from a mirror at an angle, an ultrasound beam can also *bend* when it strikes a tissue boundary at an angle.
- A *multipath artifact* is produced when some ultrasound is redirected by being bounced off a reflector while traveling through tissue. Think of a racquet ball hitting a wall to your left or right.
- As a result, it follows a longer path back to the transducer.
- The longer time of flight is interpreted as a greater distance from the transducer.
- The reflection is therefore placed *deeper* on the display.
- Furthermore, ultrasound display electronics are programmed to assume that ultrasound only travels back and forth in a straight path.
- If an outbound ultrasound is redirected in this fashion, it will also be *displaced laterally* on the display.
- Hence, a multipath artifact creates structures *deeper and more lateral* to where they truly belong.

Spieker LE, Hufschmid U, Oechslin E, et al. Double aortic and pulmonary valves: an artifact generated by ultrasound refraction. J Am Soc Echocardiogr. 2004;17:786–787.

REVERBERATION ARTIFACTS

- A comet tail artifact can be deliberately created during subcostal imaging of the tricuspid annulus.
- Closely spaced strong reflectors inside the fibrous tricuspid annulus can create multiple internal *short path* reflections.
- The reverberation distance traveled is short. The reflections are close together and do not appear spaced apart.
- Hence the continuous *flashlight beam* appearance.
- The tricuspid annulus comet tail artifacts can travel far and are often easier to see over an echo-free background such as the left atrial cavity. This may raise unwarranted concerns about a left atrial mass.
- An aortic prosthesis in the PLAX view can create a different reverberation artifact: A series of bright horizontal interrupted ladder-like arc-shaped bands appear evenly spaced. The bands get progressively weaker with distance.
- This is explained as follows:
  - There is a large acoustic impedance mismatch between the prosthesis and the surrounding tissues.
  - This sets up strong surface (not internal) reflections that try to return to the transducer surface, and get redirected right back to the valve.
  - Simply stated: The ping pong game is between the prosthesis surface and the transducer surface.
  - There are strong reflections at the same prosthesis location that keep returning to the transducer, and they get reflected right back to the prosthesis from the transducer surface.

- The process is repeated.
- There is a time delay with each successive reflection, and the reflections get progressively *weaker* due to ultrasound attenuation.
- Scanning tips with reverberation artifacts:
  - Decrease the ultrasound gain or power, and "turn the comet tail to a Venetian blind."
  - Both comet tail and ladder rung phenomena can be present in the same patient.
  - Turning down the gain may remove the relatively *weaker short path* internal reflections and preserve the stronger evenly spaced surface reflections.
  - Try turning harmonics on and off. The artifacts should be more evident with harmonics off.
  - The transducer should be manipulated to make reverberation artifacts come and go.
  - Multiple ladder-like evanescent artifacts in the PLAX ascending aorta make a dissection flap less likely.
  - See the references below and the section on lung ultrasound.

Pamnani A, Skubas NJ. Imaging artifacts during **transesophageal** echocardiography. Anesth Analg. 2014;118:516–520.

Tchelepi H, Ralls PW. **Color** comet-tail artifact: clinical applications. Am J Roentgenol. 2009;192:11–18.

Thickman DI, Ziskin MC, Goldenberg NJ, et al. Clinical manifestations of the **comet tail** artifact. J Ultrasound Med. 1983;2:225–230.

Vignon P, Spencer KT, Rambaud G, et al. Differential transesophageal echocardiographic diagnosis between linear artifacts and intraluminal flap of aortic **dissection** or disruption. Chest. 2001;119:1778–1790.

SCATTER

- Familiar mirror example of light wave scatter: When there is moisture condensation on the surface of a mirror, light is scattered instead of being reflected. Hence the blurry reflection (Fig. 1-5).
- Breast implants scatter ultrasound and create cloudy 2D images of the heart.

Movahed MR. Interference of breast implants with echocardiographic image acquisition and interpretation. Cardiovasc Ultrasound. 2007;5:9.

- When ultrasound energy is scattered in multiple directions away from the primary beam, it results in relatively *weak* returning ultrasound signals when compared with specular reflections.
- Doppler analysis of blood flow *needs* this scattered ultrasound from blood cells. This is the reason why Doppler imaging requires higher ultrasound transmission amplitudes than 2D imaging.
- Caution:
  - Higher ultrasound transmission amplitudes can destroy ultrasound contrast bubbles.

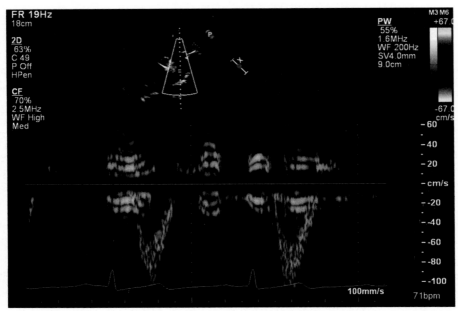

FIGURE 1-5. Stripe artifacts caused by patient talking while the descending aorta is being scanned from the suprasternal window.

- They also raise concerns about ultrasound safety.
- When imaging a fetus in utero you should use 2D imaging preferentially, and more extensively, and try to limit your use of Doppler to essential information.

SLICE THICKNESS ARTIFACT AND BEAM WIDTH ARTIFACT

- There is a misconception that the "slice" thickness of an ultrasound image is always "razor thin," small, and uniform.
- Reflections from above and from below the scanning plane can actually appear quite often in an ultrasound image.
- If a cardiac chamber is being scanned, and a solid reflection is superimposed on the cavity, there may be a false impression of an intracavitary mass or thrombus.
- A scattered reflection from a rib above or below the scanning plane frequently clouds echocardiographic images.
- A calcified sinotubular ridge or a bicuspid raphe can appear superimposed on top of the aortic leaflets in short-axis parasternal and TEE views. This can give a mistaken impression of aortic stenosis.
- Examples of beam width artifacts on the aortic valve:
  - Two side-by-side reflectors appear as one: Two small calcified nodules of Arantius on an aortic leaflet can become broadened. They may appear as a small line when they touch in diastole.
  - A small reflector such as an aortic leaflet commissure frequently appears as a line in PLAX (combined beam width and sidelobe artifact).

- A small echolucent area of an aortic root abscess can become "smeared" or filled in by reflections from neighboring solid tissue.
- The difference between slice thickness artifacts and beam width artifacts is that the anatomic structure causing a slice thickness artifact is above or below the ultrasound image. It may be visualized by rotating the transducer. Beam width artifacts distort anatomy that is already in the imaging plane.

ACOUSTIC IMPEDANCE

- This is a measure of resistance to sound passing through tissue.
- Acoustic impedance is different in tissues with different density.
- Example: Blood in the left ventricle is less dense than the ventricular walls.
- As ultrasound travels through tissue, some amount gets reflected, refracted, or scattered wherever there is a difference in acoustic impedance.
- Acoustic impedance *provides the explanation* as to how reflected ultrasound is used to recreate the anatomy of the heart. The reflections at each acoustic interface are used for echocardiographic imaging.

MATCHING LAYER

- Ultrasound transducers have a layer or more of material in front of the crystal called the matching layer.
- The purpose is to reduce acoustic mismatch between the transducer and the body.
- This reduces ultrasound reflection as ultrasound enters and exits the body.
- Gel is applied between the skin and the transducer for the same reason.

Goldstein A. Broadband **transducers** improve image quality. Diagn Imaging. 1993;15:89–93, 100.

Whittingham TA. Broadband **transducers**. Eur Radiol. 1999;9 Suppl 3:S298–S303.

NOTES

CHAPTER 2

Doppler

"Velocity: Which way and How fast?"

- The change between the pitch of transmitted sound and the pitch of received sound is used to determine direction and speed of blood cells and cardiac tissue.
- Familiar *audible sound* example of the Doppler effect: The whistle of a moving train tells you train direction and train speed.
- Historical anecdotes:
  - In 1842 Christian Doppler wrote that *light* from moving stars changes color (light frequency).
  - In 1845 the Doppler effect was scientifically validated by using *sound*:

    A note from a trumpet player on a train moving at 40 mph was perceived as a tone higher than the identical note from a stationary trumpet player.

Bullot's confirmation of Doppler's theory. In Gilllespie EC (ed): Dictionary of Scientific Biography. Vol 4. New York, NY: Charles Scribner's Sons; 1980:167.

- Other historic names in sound and ultrasound:
  - Marin Mersenne (1588–1648) studied the vibration of stretched strings.
  - Abbe Lazzaro Spallanzani (1727–1799) showed that bats navigate by echolocation.
  - Curie and Curie described the piezoelectric effect in 1880.
  - Lewis Fry Richardson registered a patent for iceberg detection using acoustic echolocation in air in April 1912. A month later he registered a similar patent for echolocation in water.
  - Paul Langevin and Constantin Chilowsky filed two U.S. patents in 1916 and 1917 for the first ultrasonic *submarine* detector using an electrostatic method (singing condenser) for one patent, and thin quartz crystals for the other. The amount of time taken by the signal to travel to the enemy submarine and echo back to the ship, on which the device was mounted, was used to calculate the distance under water.
  - S.Ya. Sokolov proposed an *acoustic microscopy* device in 1936 for producing magnified views of structures.

- Karl Theo Dussik, an Austrian neurologist, used transmitted (rather than reflected) ultrasound in 1941 to outline the ventricles of the human brain.
- W. D. Keidel used ultrasound in 1950 to examine the heart. He transmitted ultrasonic waves through the heart and recorded the effect of ultrasound on the *other side* of the chest. His purpose was to measure cardiac volumes.
- Helmut Hertz obtained a commercial ultrasonoscope in 1953. It was being used for nondestructive material testing. It was based on the work of Floyd Firestone, who applied for a U.S. invention patent in 1940.
- Hertz collaborated with Inge Edler, a cardiologist in Sweden. They used this commercial ultrasonoscope to examine the heart. This is considered by many as the beginning of echocardiography.
- In the early 1960s, investigators in Shanghai and Wuhan began with an A-mode ultrasound device, and then developed an M-mode recorder. They described fetal echocardiography, and contrast echocardiography.

Coman IM, Popescu BA. Shigeo Satomura: 60 years of **Doppler** ultrasound in medicine. Cardiovasc Ultrasound. 2015;13:48.

Curie P, Curie J. Developpement, par pression de l'electricite polaire dans les cristaux hemiedres a faces inclines. Comptes Rendus. 1880;91:291–295.

Curie P, Curie J. Lois du degagement de l'electricite par pression, dans la tourmaline. Comptes Rendus. 1881;92:186–188.

Edler I. The diagnostic use of ultrasound in heart disease. Acta Med Scand Suppl. 1955;308:32.

Edler I. Ultrasound cardiogram in mitral valve disease. Acta Chir Scand. 1956;111:230.

Edler I, Hertz CH. Use of ultrasonic reflectoscope for the continuous recording of movements of heart walls. Kungl Fysiogr Sallsk Lung Forth. 1954;24:40.

Feigenbaum H. Evolution of echocardiography. Circulation. 1996;93:1321–1327.

Feigenbaum H, Waldhausen JA, Hyde LP. Ultrasound diagnosis of pericardial effusion. JAMA. 1965;191:711–714.

Franklin DL, Schlegel W, Rushmer RF. Blood flow measured by Doppler frequency shift of back-scattered ultrasound. Science. 1961;134:564–565.

Hatle L, Angelsen B, Tromsdal A. Noninvasive assessment of aortic stenosis by Doppler ultrasound. Br Heart J. 1980;43:284–292.

Hsu CC. Ultrasonic diagnostics. Shang Sci Tech Press. 1961;167.

Joyner CR Jr, Reid JM, Bond JP. Reflected ultrasound in the assessment of mitral valve disease. Circulation. 1963;27:503–511.

Kaneko Z. First steps in the development of the Doppler flowmeter. Ultrasound Med Biol. 1986;12:187–195.

Keidel WD. Uber eine Methode zur Registrierung der Volumanderungen des Herzens am Menschen. Z Kreislaufforsch. 1950;39:257.

Miller DC. An Anecdotal History of the Science of Sound. New York, NY: Macmillan; 1935.

Peronneau P, Deloche A, Bui-Mong-Hung, et al. Ultrasonic flowmetry—developments and experimental applications. Eur Surg Res. 1969;1:147–156.

Roelandt JR. Seeing the invisible: a short history of cardiac ultrasound. Eur J Echocardiogr. 2000;1:8–11.

Veyrat C. Daniel Kalmanson, pioneer of **intracardiac** Doppler exploration in 1969: Emphasis on the first mitral and tricuspid flow velocity recordings. Ultrasound Med Biol. 2006;32:783–789.

Veyrat C. The glorious years leading Doppler flow to the heart, the odyssey of the pioneers! Acta Cardiol. 2014;69:351–365.

Wang XF, Xiso JP, et al. **Fetal** echocardiography—method for pregnancy diagnosis. Chin J Obstet Gynecol. 1964;10:267–269.

Wild PW. **Early history** of echocardiography. J Cardiovasc Ultrasonogr. 1996;5:2.

AUDIO DEPICTION OF FREQUENCY SHIFT

"Why do I hear sound when ultrasound studies are being performed?"

- Although clinical ultrasound uses MHz frequencies, the change between transmitted and received frequencies is relatively small, and is often in the range of audible sound frequencies under 20,000 Hz. This allows an audio output of the frequency *shift* to the speaker of an ultrasound device. The operator can use the audible pitch to determine optimal beam angle, and to establish presence of turbulent blood flow (harsh rather than musical audio).

FREQUENCY SHIFT TO SPECTRAL DISPLAY

- The frequency shift is translated by the Doppler equation to the familiar Doppler spectral display of velocities.
- In other words, sound frequency (Hz) is converted to speed and direction (cm/s toward, or away from the transducer). When speed has a direction, it is called velocity.
- This conversion is performed instantly by the ultrasound machine. As a result, the Doppler equation is never directly manipulated or calculated by the operator.
- Note: Quite often in quick echo lab conversations about Doppler information, we catch ourselves wrongly talking about frequency when we actually mean frequency *shift*. In a Doppler-related discussion it is quicker (but incorrect) to say "frequency" rather than the correct "change in frequency."

THE DOPPLER EQUATION

- It is important to note that the calculation above is affected by the ultrasound frequency being used for imaging.
- In addition, the Doppler formula calculation assumes that the angle of blood or cardiac tissue movement being measured is *parallel* to the ultrasound beam.
- Ultrasound machines have angle of incidence correction capabilities that are adjustable by the sonographer.
- The mathematical technique that separates the spectrum of frequency shifts into individual components for the Doppler equation is called the *fast Fourier transform*. This is similar to the way a musical chord can be expressed in terms of the amplitudes and frequencies of its constituent notes.

PULSED DOPPLER

- Pulsed-wave Doppler displays blood flow speed, blood flow direction, and signal amplitude.
- Medical imaging ultrasound does not "ring like a church bell." When the user turns on pulsed Doppler, the transducer emits bursts of ultrasound "clicks" that return to the transducer with frequency shift information.
- Some blind people have mastered the skill of emitting clicks with their mouth to judge distance of surrounding, sound-reflective structures such as walls.

- Pulsed Doppler allows *range gating*: It is possible for the user to select an area of interest in the body and limit the Doppler analysis to a set distance from the transducer.
- The machine calculates the time of flight back and forth from the area of interest. It only listens for the returning ultrasound at the appropriate time.
- Practical example: It is possible to obtain Doppler information from the left ventricular outflow without "contaminating" it with other nearby flow velocities from the mitral or aortic valves.
- Excessive range gating *distances* create a sampling error artifact: aliasing.
- Familiar cinema phenomenon that illustrates aliasing:
  - Airplane propellers, or wagon wheels seemingly changing speed, or turning in the wrong direction in a movie are due to a video frame rate sampling error ("Nyquist frequency").
  - Aliasing is a consequence of a sampling rate that is too slow.
  - Deeper sampling reduces sampling rate (listening time is longer).
  - Lower-frequency transducers permit lower sampling rates before aliasing happens.
- Pulsed-wave Doppler imaging caveats:
  - Know how to adjust the *range gate* size to maximize the desired signal, and to minimize the noise.
  - Adjust the baseline up or down to maximize the desired signal. Fill the screen with the signal that shows the desired direction.
  - Adjust the baseline wall filter according to the desired signal. Don't filter out important low-velocity signals. Example: Patent foramen ovale is a low-velocity signal.
  - Adjust the sweep speed: Fast sweeps for measurements, slow sweeps for respiratory changes.
  - Align the Doppler beam in parallel with the blood flow or tissue movement.
  - Use the lowest possible ultrasound frequencies.
  - Get as close as possible to the area of interest.

ULTRASOUND CLICKS

- Familiar hotel check-in example:
  - When you ring a bell to summon the bellhop, there is a long pleasant musical tone composed of "a narrow range of frequencies with their harmonic multiples."
  - If you *dampen* the ringing by placing your hand on the bell, there is a short muffled click.
  - Ultrasound imaging transducers are dampened.
  - A click is less pleasant to the ear because it has a broader range of frequencies.
  - A click is a form of static-like noise (nonmusical, harsh, broad-frequency noise). The nonharmonic frequencies of a click are clustered around the fundamental frequency of the bell or transducer.

- A broader range of frequencies is also called increased frequency *bandwidth*.
- Tuning forks exemplify the opposite: A narrow bandwidth.

BANDWIDTH AND GAIN SETTINGS IN PULSED-WAVE DOPPLER

- The "clicks" of pulsed-wave Doppler have a *variable* bandwidth of frequencies:
  - Shorter pulses have a wider bandwidth.
  - Longer pulses have a narrower bandwidth.
- Narrower bandwidth improves the ability to detect a *weak* Doppler shift signal.
- Gain can be increased by the operator to *amplify* weak signals.
- Increased gain affects the signal to noise ratio.
- As ultrasound travels through tissue, the higher bandwidth frequencies become attenuated to a greater degree than the lower bandwidth frequencies.
- The preferential attenuation of higher bandwidth frequencies may be misinterpreted by the ultrasound machine as a Doppler shift.
- Think of the above principles when adjusting:
  - Doppler gain.
  - Pulsed-wave Doppler gate size.
  - Transducer distance to area of interest.

PULSED-WAVE DOPPLER TERMINOLOGY

- This is what true echocardiographers think about while hitting a *tennis ball against a wall*.
- The following is a lengthy and contrived *visual* tennis racquet metaphor for pulsed Doppler ultrasound. It is intended to introduce ultrasound terminology.
- Standing in front of a wall, sending a ball at the wall at a *uniform* velocity— average speed of ultrasound through tissue is a *uniform* 1540 m/s.
- Making note of the strength of the returning impact *intensity*.
- *Comparing* the returning impact to the throw ("frequency" *shift* that generates Doppler information).
- The time it takes the ball to travel back and forth changes with the distance from the wall (*pulse repetition period*). In echo, "time is distance."
- It is unfortunately necessary to wait for the impact information while the ball is in motion (i.e., ultrasound travels through tissue).
- The *rate* of listening for the ultrasound to return is the pulse repetition frequency.
- The *time* spent listening is the pulse repetition period.
- In ultrasound scanning, there is no flying tennis ball to watch. The waiting transducer can only make assumptions about what is happening.
- During the time spent waiting, the "deaf and blind" ultrasound system is programmed to make the following *assumptions* about what is happening during back-and-forth ultrasound wave propagation:

- Ultrasound travels only in straight lines parallel to the central transducer beam.
- Anatomic structures only reflect an ultrasound beam once.
- Reflections are only from structures directly in the path of the beam.
- The position of a structure is proportional to ultrasound travel time.
- Note: Wrong violated assumptions cause imaging *artifacts*.

RANGE AMBIGUITY—HPRF DOPPLER

- A metaphoric "tennis robot with a computer" (multigated multipulse Doppler) can get more (frequency shift) information by throwing multiple sequential balls (high pulse repetition frequency, or HPRF), but this may also create *wrong* information (aliasing, range ambiguity) by confusing the multiple metaphoric balls that are simultaneously traveling in the metaphoric air.
- There are also multiple metaphoric bumpy complicated *walls*—ultrasound travels and scatters through multiple layers of tissue with variable reflectivity creating a spectrum of frequency shifts. See the section on acoustic impedance.
- 2D range (distance) *ambiguity* from multiple reflectors:
  - Sound is reflected from multiple sequential mountain ranges, but it is not clear which echo is coming from which mountain range: This happens if you "yodel" a second time before the first set of echoes dies out.
  - If a delayed ultrasound echo from a previous transducer pulse returns to the transducer *after* a new pulse went out, the transducer may wrongly interpret the old reflection as a reflection from the newer pulse. As a result, ultrasound information from deep structures is *wrongly placed* with information from shallow structures.
- HPRF Doppler does not wait for a Doppler signal to return. It creates range ambiguity to overcome Nyquist limitations.
- Two examples of 2D range ambiguity:
  - A pleural effusion may allow ultrasound to travel far past the heart before being reflected. Delayed echoes returning from these distances to the transducer confuse the machine electronics, and hazy arc-like reflections can get displayed on top of normal cardiac anatomy.
  - Imaging the apical region of the left ventricle at a shallow depth (looking for a thrombus) allows for rapid firing of transmit pulses. Delayed reflections from previous pulses create blurry near field artifacts because the ultrasound system cannot distinguish reflections of old pulses from new pulses.

Baker DW, Rubenstein SA, Lorch GS. **Pulsed Doppler** echocardiography: principles and applications. Am J Med. 1977;63: 69–80.

Bom K, de Boo J, Rijsterborgh H. On the **aliasing** problem in pulsed Doppler cardiac studies. J Clin Ultrasound. 1984;12: 559–567.

Gill RW, Kossoff MB, Kossoff G, et al. New class of pulsed Doppler US **ambiguity** at short ranges. Radiology. 1989;173: 272–275.

Moss CF, Surlykke A. Auditory scene analysis by **echolocation** in bats. J Acoust Soc Am. 2001;110:2207–2226.

MIRROR ARTIFACT IN PULSED-WAVE DOPPLER

- This is a common artifact that is fixable to some degree by:
  - Reducing Doppler gain.
  - Adjusting the ultrasound beam angle closer to parallel to flow (zero degrees).
- A mirrored "ghost" pulsed-wave Doppler signal is displayed in the opposite direction of real flow.
- Usually the amplitude (brightness) of the displayed mirror signal is weaker than the amplitude of the real flow display.
- This is caused at the *directional separating circuits* on the echo machine, resulting in incomplete separation between the forward and reverse channels.
- It is affected by the *angle* of insonation: When the ultrasound beam angle approaches an unworkable 90 degrees to flow, part of the reflection is assigned to the wrong directional circuit.

SPECTRAL BROADENING IN PULSED-WAVE DOPPLER

- When blood flow is laminar, there is a narrow range of Doppler flow shifts. The Doppler display is a narrow band of velocities with an echo-free area "under the curve."
- Turbulent blood flow manifests as spectral broadening with *loss* of this echo-free area. The pulsed-wave signal resembles a continuous wave signal.
- On tracing the Doppler signal envelope, the *outer edge* should be used.
- Terminology: The brightest part of a pulsed-wave Doppler signal envelope is known as the *modal* velocity. Do not trace on top of the modal velocity. Trace the outer edge.

Kyranis SJ, Latona J, Platts D, et al. Improving the echocardiographic assessment of pulmonary pressure using the tricuspid regurgitant signal—The "chin" vs the "beard". Echocardiography. 2018;35:1085–1096.

When tracing the outer edge—avoid the noise. Give the noisy Doppler envelope a "haircut".

TISSUE DOPPLER

- The velocity of myocardium (rather than the velocity of blood) can be measured with Doppler after adjusting instrument gain and filter settings. Tissue velocity signals are *stronger and slower* than blood cell signals.
- Tissue Doppler plays a key role in estimating left atrial pressures.
- Tissue Doppler from two points in the myocardium can determine strain and strain rate.

Abudiab MM, Schutt RC, Kumar A, et al. Estimating left ventricular **filling pressure** by echocardiography. J Am Coll Cardiol. 2017;69:1937–1948.

Mitter SS, Shah SJ, Thomas JD. A test in context: E/A and E/e' to assess diastolic dysfunction and LV filling pressure. J Am Coll Cardiol. 2017;69:1451–1464.

Mor-Avi V, Lang RM, Badano LP, et al. Current and evolving echocardiographic techniques for the quantitative evaluation of **cardiac mechanics**. J Am Soc Echocardiogr. 2011;24:277–313.

Nagueh SF, Middleton KJ, Kopelen HA, et al. Doppler tissue imaging: a noninvasive technique for evaluation of left ventricular relaxation and estimation of **filling pressures**. J Am Coll Cardiol. 1997;30:1527–1533.

Sohn DW, Chai IH, Lee DJ, et al. Assessment of **mitral annulus** velocity by Doppler tissue imaging in the evaluation of left ventricular diastolic function. J Am Coll Cardiol. 1997;30:474–480.

WALL FILTERS

- The pulsed-wave Doppler display is intended to show speed and direction of red blood cells.
- Unfortunately, much stronger undesirable Doppler signals get created by valves, cardiac motion, respiration, etc.
- Fortunately, the velocities of these strong signals are *slower* than the desired red blood cell velocities. The slow velocities of the strong undesirable signals can be filtered out.
- A wall filter permits the desired high blood flow velocities to be displayed while rejecting low-velocity baseline noise.
- If a wall filter setting is too low, Doppler circuits may become saturated by noise and rendered ineffective.
- The displayed result of applying a wall filter is a *black band* around the pulsed-wave Doppler baseline.

SCANNING TIPS

- Wall filters should be adjusted in conjunction with the dynamic range controls to allow the range of desired blood flow velocities to be displayed.
- During 3D color flow imaging of mitral regurgitation, it may be useful to turn the wall filters up to isolate and localize the high-velocity components of the mitral regurgitation jet.

DOPPLER EQUATION AND TRANSDUCER FREQUENCY

Doppler frequency shift = 2 × speed of blood (or speed of tissue) × transducer frequency × angle of incidence (see cosine discussion below) ÷ propagation speed through the tissue (1540 m/s)

- Transducer frequency:
  - As transducer frequency increases, frequency *shift* from the same blood motion, or tissue motion, increases as well.
- Technical implication:
  - Manually switching an ultrasound transducer affects returning ultrasound frequencies. Switching to a smaller size, higher-frequency transducer will provide higher returning frequencies from the same structures.
  - After changing transducers, there may be no evident change of displayed Doppler velocities to the sonographer, because the machine immediately uses the Doppler equation to recalculate the returning ultrasound information based on the new transducer frequency.

en.wikipedia.org/wiki/Über_das_farbige_Licht_der_Doppelsterne_und_einiger_anderer_Gestirne_des_Himmels

Annotated Wikipedia summary of Christian Doppler's treatise: "On the colored light of the binary stars and some other stars of the heavens."

COSINE

"A trigonometry calculation that corrects for an existing angle between the transmitted sound beam, and the direction of blood, or tissue movement."

- When the angle is 0, cosine is 1; angle adjustment is not needed.
- When the angle is 90, cosine is 0; Doppler shift cannot be calculated.
- In practice, the angle should be kept well under 30 degrees.

CONTINUOUS-WAVE DOPPLER

- Ultrasound is constantly transmitted (duty factor is 1.0 [100%]).
- *All* returning ultrasound signals are converted to velocities by the ultrasound machine using the Doppler equation (range ambiguity).
- The returning velocities are overlapped on the cardiac cycle display.
- This is necessary for high Doppler velocities (aortic stenosis, mitral regurgitation, ventricular septal defect, pulmonary hypertension).
- There is no time gain compensation. The TGC sliders don't work. *Overall* gain has to be adjusted.
- Signals from *deeper* blood or tissue movements are *weaker* than more shallow signals.
- Therefore, a *weak* signal does not necessarily mean that *fewer* red blood cells are responsible.
- This is an important concept to keep in mind when evaluating severity of valvular regurgitation.

COLOR FLOW DOPPLER

- Color flow Doppler is a spatial display of velocities in real time.
- It is superimposed on 2D information.
- Doppler information is encoded into colors.
- The colors give direction and speed of either blood cells or cardiac muscle.
- Color hues display gradation of velocities (red is slower than yellow, blue is slower than white).
- Each color grade corresponds to a mean blood flow velocity.

Aggarwal KK, Moos S, Philpot EF, et al. Color velocity determination using pixel color intensity in Doppler color flow mapping. Echocardiography. 1989;6:473–483.

Miyatake K, Okamoto M, Kinoshita N, et al. Clinical applications of a new type of real-time two-dimensional Doppler flow imaging system. Am J Cardiol. 1984;54:857–868.

Pozniak MA, Zagzebski JA, Scanlan KA. Spectral and color Doppler **artifacts**. Radiographics. 1992;12:35–44.

Color Doppler Packets

- Simply put, a color Doppler image is created by repeated Doppler evaluation of bunches of single repeating lines of ultrasound called packets.

- Adjacent acoustic packet lines are combined like a 2D image to create a two-dimensional color display of Doppler information (which way, how fast).
- The color bar on the display provides a reference scale of *mean* velocity.
- Technical suggestion for setting color gain:
  - Increase the gain until noise pixels appear, and then lower the gain just slightly to make them disappear. This brings out weak signals and prevents overgaining.
  - Overgaining creates an exaggerated, potentially misleading, color flow display that "bleeds" into adjacent areas.

COLOR FLOW ARTIFACTS

- **Aliasing:**
  - Color reversal at the point that the Nyquist limit is reached.
  - Flow in one direction is *wrongly* assigned a potentially misleading color, wrongly indicating flow in the opposite direction.
- Practical scanning points to decrease aliasing:
  - Position the transducer to scan *closer* to the area of interest.
  - Use a *lower* transducer frequency.
  - Move the *baseline* to increase the velocity range in the desired direction (used in PISA calculation).
- **Mirror Artifact:**
  - False duplication of a color flow image.
  - Due to ultrasound interaction with a strong reflector.
  - The mirror image is displayed upside-down on the other side of the reflector.
- **Color Ghosting:**
  - Brief flashes of color on the display that do not correspond to real Doppler information.
  - Two-dimensional structures may briefly get assigned color (instead of grayscale) pixels.
  - Simplified explanation: The computer is supposed to assign grayscale pixels to relatively slow structures, and color pixels to relatively faster structures. Normal breathing or talking while being scanned may scatter ultrasound and create this artifact.
- **Missing Color:**
  - Shadowing by a prosthetic valve or by a calcified mitral annulus is a common finding.
  - Color may also be absent where there is obvious flow, due to low gain settings.

SCANNING TIP

- Color may be absent if the scale is not decreased at a foramen ovale, or at a pulmonary vein ostium.

- **Directional Ambiguity:**

  This is a common confusing color flow finding when imaging the aorta with flow 90 degrees to the transducer:

  - Flow approaching the scan lines is coded in one color.
  - Flow away from the scan lines in coded in the opposite color.
  - Half the vessel is red and half the vessel is blue.

COLOR BAR

- In contrast to pulsed-flow Doppler, the color bar does not display Doppler signal amplitude (strength). Weak and strong Doppler signals with the same frequency shift are assigned the same pixel color.
- The black band in the middle of the bar indicates the velocity below which color flow is filtered out and not displayed. Color flow displays of blood velocities assign low *tissue* velocities to the black band.
- The numbers on the top and bottom indicate the highest detectable mean velocity.

PERSISTENCE SETTINGS

- Persistence is a frame-to-frame averaging "image smoothing" technique.
- Turning off persistence will result in an unprocessed raw 2D image that may sometimes appear unnaturally grainy.
- Keeping persistence on may yield a *smoother* 2D look by averaging sequential images.
- Caution:
  - Excessive persistence may create *blurry* 2D images.
  - Excessive persistence with color flow may misrepresent the *timing and duration* of Doppler flow signals.

VARIANCE

- Green pixels are sometimes used to demonstrate variance on color flow.
- Variance is an indicator of *turbulent* rather than laminar flow.
- Color flow smoothing (persistence) may need to be turned off.

Baxter GM, Polak J. **Variance** mapping in colour flow imaging: what does it measure? Clin Radiol. 1994;49:262–265.

TEMPORAL AND SPATIAL RESOLUTION

- Frame rate (Table 2-1) and line density can be manually adjusted on an ultrasound machine. When one goes up, the other goes down (unless you change image sector size).
- Narrowing the image sector size improves both frame rate and line density.

TABLE 2-1 • Methods to Increase Frame Rate

- Decreasing image depth.
- Narrowing the width of the image sector.
- Using *preprocessing* zoom.
- Decreasing the number of focal zones.
- Reducing the number of scan lines per sector.

- Temporal resolution: A high *frame rate* should theoretically be more appropriate to visualize small, fast-moving structures such as a Lambl excrescence or a small vegetation.
- Spatial resolution: A high *line density* provides more detail in slower-moving structures. For example, a speckled "ground glass" appearance of hypertrophic myocardium may be more obvious.
- Familiar camera example: You photograph sports action using high frame rates. You photograph still flower close-ups, or portraits, using high lens apertures for better detail (line density).

TRANSDUCER FOCUS

- A transducer can be manually focused by turning a knob on the machine.
- The focal point is the narrowest area of an ultrasound beam.
- Just like in a camera lens, the focal point is expected to provide the best resolution.
- Structures that are proximal or distal to the focal point may be more blurry.

SCANNING TIPS

- The focal point should be constantly adjusted during a study—to the depth where structures of interest are located.
- For example, focusing on a difficult-to-image pulmonic valve in the short-axis view, and then moving the focus deeper toward the sometimes elusive tricuspid valve when imaging in the apical views.

- The width and spacing of individual ultrasound beams is affected by moving the focal point.
- If an ultrasound beam is narrow enough to fit between two anatomic structures, the ultrasound reflections return to the transducer at *different sweep times*, and are displayed as separate structures.
- A beam that is too wide bounces back to the transducer at the same time from adjacent structures, making them appear falsely connected.
  - Example: Nodules of Arantius on adjacent aortic leaflets can appear as a single line instead of as two separate dots when they touch in diastole.
  - Think about beam width artifacts when adjusting the focus. They are least likely at the focal point.

CHAPTER 3

Echocardiographic Quantification

2015 GUIDELINES

Lang RM, Badano LP, Mor-Avi V, et al. Recommendations for cardiac chamber quantification by echocardiography in adults. Eur Heart J Cardiovasc Imaging. 2015;16:233–270.

- Echocardiographic measurements are standardized and extensively illustrated.
- Normal values are provided.
- Calculations are explained.
- The right ventricle is included.
- Measurement criteria of the proximal ascending aorta are illustrated.

DOPPLER CALCULATIONS

- Stroke volume is calculated as the volume of a cylinder.
- The volume of a cylinder is calculated as the area of the base × height.
- Example: Left ventricular outflow stroke volume = LVOT area × LVOT VTI.
- LVOT VTI is the stroke distance (cylinder height).
- Stroke volume × heart rate = cardiac output.
- Stroke volume = end-diastolic volume × ejection fraction.
- Cardiac output = heart rate × stroke volume.
- Cardiac output = heart rate × end-diastolic volume × ejection fraction.
- Corollary:
  - Cardiac output is affected by changes in heart rate, by end diastolic volume (preload), and by ejection fraction.

- Practical clinical value: 2D echo provides a look at the impact of preload in patients with Doppler evidence of constriction, restriction, etc., by showing right and left ventricular end-diastolic volumes.

*Hurrell DG, Nishimura RA, Ilstrup DM, et al. Utility of **preload** alteration in assessment of left ventricular filling pressure by Doppler echocardiography: a simultaneous catheterization and Doppler echocardiographic study. J Am Coll Cardiol. 1997;30:459–467.*

CARDIAC OUTPUT IN THE CATH LAB

Fick Versus Thermodilution

- The *Fick* method uses the a-v O_2 difference. It works in atrial fibrillation because "steady state" is used. It is most accurate in low-output states where there is a wide a-v O_2 difference. Oxygen extraction is greater with decreased cardiac output. This results in a low pulmonary artery saturation. Pulmonary artery saturation <65% indicates decreased cardiac output.
- *Thermodilution* measures the "area under the curve" after a short set of cardiac cycles. It is less reliable in low-output states. The calculation is affected by significant tricuspid regurgitation, and possibly by the variable cardiac cycle length in atrial fibrillation.

Gonzalez J, Delafosse C, Fartoukh M, et al. Comparison of bedside measurement of cardiac output with the thermodilution method and the Fick method in mechanically ventilated patients. Crit Care. 2003;7:171–178.

DERIVATIONS FROM STROKE VOLUME CALCULATIONS

- Aortic stenosis area calculation by continuity:
  - Because of flow continuity and conservation of mass: Stroke volume is the same below the stenotic aortic valve and the same at the stenosis.
  - In other words, the stroke volume "cylinder" simply *changes* from "short and fat" to "long and thin."
  - The volume of both cylinders is identical.
- The two cylinders have a total of four components.
- If three components are known, it is possible to use a simple formula to solve for the fourth unknown component.
  Example: Calculation of aortic stenosis area by continuity.
  1. Short $\times$ *fat* = *long* $\times$ thin ("thin" is aortic stenosis orifice area).
  2. Thin = (short $\times$ *fat*) ÷ *long*.
- The four components change according to flow and degree of stenosis.
- Theoretically, in the absence of significant regurgitation, stenotic aortic valve area can be calculated by stroke volume from *anywhere* in the heart $\times$ aortic stenosis VTI.
- Shunts: Can theoretically be calculated by comparing stroke volumes.
- Regurgitation: Valvular regurgitation volumes can be calculated by simple subtraction of affected and unaffected stroke volumes.

Burns PN. *The physical principles of Doppler and spectral analysis. J Clin Ultrasound. 1987;15:567–590.*

Chafizadeh ER, Zoghbi WA. *Doppler echocardiographic assessment of the St. Jude Medical prosthetic valve in the aortic position using the continuity equation. Circulation. 1991;83:213–223.*

A Doppler velocity index, the ratio of peak velocity in the left ventricular outflow to that of the aortic jet, averaged 0.41 ± 0.09 and was less dependent on valve size (r = 0.43). Thus, the continuity equation can be applied to the assessment of prosthetic St. Jude valves in the aortic position.

Hill JC, Palma RA. *Doppler tissue imaging for the assessment of left ventricular diastolic function: a systematic approach for the sonographer. J Am Soc Echocardiogr. 2005;18:80–88.*

Ho CY, Solomon SD. *A clinician's guide to tissue Doppler imaging. Circulation. 2006;113:e396–e398.*

Nagueh SF, Sun H, Kopelen HA, et al. *Hemodynamic determinants of the mitral annulus diastolic velocities by tissue Doppler. J Am Coll Cardiol. 2001;37:278–285.*

Nikitin NP, Witte KK, Thackray SD, et al. *Longitudinal ventricular function: normal values of atrioventricular annular and myocardial velocities measured with quantitative two-dimensional color Doppler tissue imaging. J Am Soc Echocardiogr. 2003;16:906–921.*

Waggoner AD, Bierig SM. *Tissue Doppler imaging: a useful echocardiographic method for the cardiac sonographer to assess systolic and diastolic ventricular function. J Am Soc Echocardiogr. 2001;14:1143–1152.*

SIMPLIFIED BERNOULLI EQUATION

- Doppler velocity is used to determine pressure gradients.
- Pressure differences in cardiac chambers can be calculated from Doppler measurements of blood flow velocities. Pressure difference = $4V^2$
- Pressure gradient calculations are used extensively in adult and pediatric cardiology.
- Examples:
  - Aortic stenosis.
  - Pulmonic stenosis.
  - Right ventricular end-diastolic pressure (from PI jet).
  - Left ventricular end-diastolic pressure (from AI jet).
  - Interventricular gradients.
  - Coarctation gradients.

Question: *Where* **is the lowest pressure in aortic valve stenosis?**

Answer: Just past the stenotic aortic valve, where the velocity is the highest.

- This is important for understanding pressure recovery, and for keeping your distance from the aortic valve when performing pulsed-wave Doppler interrogation of the left ventricular outflow tract.

AORTIC VALVE AREA CALCULATION IN THE CATH LAB

- The valve area can be calculated in the cath lab by the simple *Hakki* formula:
  - Cardiac output is divided by the square root of the gradient across the aortic valve.

Hakki AH, Iskandrian AS, Bemis CE, et al. *A simplified valve formula for the calculation of stenotic cardiac valve areas. Circulation. 1981;63:1050–1055.*

- *A simplified version of the original Gorlin formula using the cardiac output and the pressure difference across the valve can be used to measure the severity of aortic stenosis.*
- **Peak** pressure difference across the valve can be used instead of the mean pressure difference.
- Pitfall of *echocardiographic* aortic stenosis calculation: The left ventricular outflow diameter can be overestimated or underestimated, giving an incorrect stroke volume.
- In theory, two diameters are better than one: Since the shape of the left ventricular outflow resembles an ellipse, two diameters obtained by 3D can be used to calculate the elliptical left ventricular outflow area as follows:
  - Area of an ellipse = $(\pi \div 4) \times$ (diameter one) $\times$ (diameter two).
- Cath-echo discrepancy of aortic valve area may be due to pressure recovery, as discussed in the two references below.

Baumgartner H, Khan S, DeRobertis M, et al. **Discrepancies** between Doppler and catheter gradients in aortic prosthetic valves in vitro: a manifestation of localized gradients and pressure recovery. Circulation. 1990;82:1467–1475.

Chambers J. Is pressure recovery an important cause of "Doppler aortic stenosis" with no gradient at cardiac catheterisation? Heart. 1996;76:381–383.

PRESSURE, FLOW, AND RESISTANCE

- Flow is determined by pressure difference and by resistance.
- Familiar garden hose example:
  - By putting your thumb on a garden hose, you create variable *resistance*.
  - By turning the spigot, you create variable *flow* from the higher pressure plumbing to the lower pressure hose.
- Flow velocity is a form of *kinetic* energy.
- Pressure is a form of *potential* energy.
- Potential energy is the *stored ability* to create flow by being able to overcome resistance.
- Energy can change from potential to kinetic and back, but the total amount of energy is conserved.
- When energy is conserved and not dissipated as heat, the sum of potential and kinetic energy in a particular location remains the same.

OHM'S LAW

- Resistance = Pressure $\div$ Flow.
- Pressure = Resistance $\times$ Flow.
- Atrial septal defect example: Pulmonary artery pressure will increase with increased resistance in the pulmonary vascular bed, and with increased flow into the pulmonary vascular bed through a left to right shunt.
- Flow = Pressure $\div$ Resistance.
- Flow decreases as resistance increases.

- Wikipedia reading assignments:
  - Pressure–volume loop analysis in cardiology.
  - Wiggers diagram.
  - Cardiovascular physiology.
  - Fick principle.
  - Cardiac output.

DOPPLER DERIVATION OF RESISTANCE

- Flow = Area × TVI × HR.
- Flow = Δ Pressure ÷ Resistance.
- Resistance = Δ Pressure ÷ Area × TVI × HR.
- Δ Pressure = $4V^2$.
- Resistance = $4V^2$ ÷ Area × TVI × HR.

*Abbas AE, Fortuin FD, Schiller NB, et al. A **simple method** for noninvasive estimation of pulmonary vascular resistance. J Am Coll Cardiol. 2003;41:1021–1027.*

- *Peak tricuspid regurgitant velocity / right ventricular outflow tract time-velocity integral.*
- *A cutoff value of 0.175 had a sensitivity of 77% and a specificity of 81% for pulmonary vascular resistance >2 Wood units.*

*Kaga S, Mikami T, Murayama M, et al. A **new method** to estimate pulmonary vascular resistance using diastolic pulmonary artery–right ventricular pressure gradients derived from continuous wave Doppler velocity measurements of pulmonary regurgitation. Int J Cardiovasc Imaging. 2017;33:31–38. (See Fig. 3-1.)*

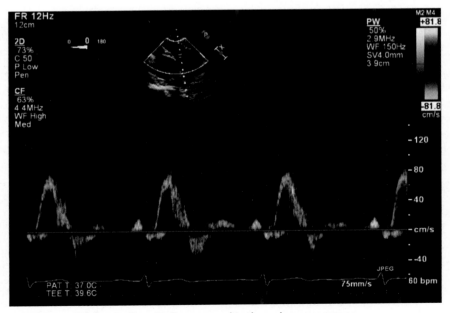

FIGURE 3-1. Brief early diastolic flow reversal in the pulmonary artery.

- *The difference between the Doppler-derived early-diastolic and end-diastolic pulmonary artery (PA)–right ventricular (RV) pressure gradients divided by the cardiac output (measured in the left ventricular outflow tract by echocardiography).*

POISEUILLE'S LAW

- Pressure increases as blood flow volume increases.
- Pressure increases as blood vessel caliber *decreases.*
- Resistance increases as blood vessel caliber decreases.

CALCULATING RIGHT VENTRICULAR SYSTOLIC PRESSURE

- The Bernoulli equation is used with the peak tricuspid regurgitation velocity to calculate the gradient across the tricuspid valve.
- The right ventricular systolic pressure (RVSP) is calculated as the sum of this peak gradient plus the estimated right atrial pressure.
- Advanced concepts:
  - Right ventricular systolic function, tricuspid annulus dilatation, decreased tricuspid leaflet coaptation, and right atrial compliance all may affect TR velocity.
  - Caution: RVSP = PASP (pulmonary artery systolic pressure) only in absence of pulmonic valve stenosis, or other forms of right ventricular outflow obstruction.

Question: In the presence of pulmonic valve stenosis, there may be pressure recovery. Should you use *peak* or *mean* PS gradient?

Answer: Mean (see references below).

Berger M, Haimowitz A, Van Tosh A, et al. Quantitative assessment of pulmonary hypertension in patients with tricuspid regurgitation using continuous wave Doppler ultrasound. J Am Coll Cardiol. 1985;6:359–365.

Parasuraman S, Walker S, Loudon BL, et al. Assessment of pulmonary artery pressure by echocardiography—a **comprehensive review**. Int J Cardiol Heart Vasc. 2016;12:45–51.

Silvilairat S, Cabalka AK, Cetta F, et al. Echocardiographic assessment of isolated **pulmonary valve stenosis**: which outpatient Doppler gradient has the most clinical validity? J Am Soc Echocardiogr. 2005;18:1137–1142.

Yock PG, Popp RL. Noninvasive estimation of right ventricular systolic pressure by Doppler ultrasound in patients with tricuspid regurgitation. Circulation. 1984;70:657–662.

DIASTOLIC AND MEAN PULMONARY ARTERY PRESSURE

- Elevated pulmonary artery pressure may be due to:
  - Increased flow.
  - Increased resistance.
- Resistance can be estimated by the ratio of peak TR velocity ÷ PA velocity time integral.
- End-diastolic pulmonary regurgitation gradient (EDPR) is a correlate of pulmonary artery *diastolic* pressure.

- It suggests abnormal hemodynamics when >5 mm Hg.
- EDPR gradient may exceed 10 or even 15 mm Hg, strongly indicating elevated pulmonary artery diastolic pressure.
- Three methods to measure *mean* pulmonary artery pressure:
  - Peak (opening) pulmonic regurgitation gradient.
  - Planimetry of the tricuspid regurgitation signal.
  - The formula used for calculating mean arterial systolic pressure (mean pressure = [systole + 2 diastole] ÷ 3) may be applied if diastolic pressure from EDPR is available.

Schiller NB, Ristow B. Doppler under pressure: it's time to cease the folly of chasing the peak right ventricular systolic pressure. J Am Soc Echocardiogr. 2013;26:479–482.

THE FLYING W

- Mid-systolic flow deceleration and notching of right ventricular outflow velocities is the Doppler equivalent of the old "Flying W" M-mode sign—mid-systolic closure of the pulmonic valve (Fig. 3-2).
- It is considered an indicator of elevated pulmonary vascular *resistance*.

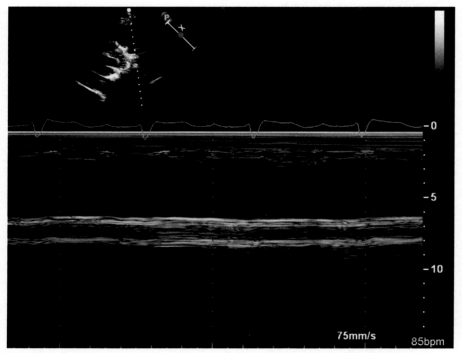

FIGURE 3-2. Mid-systolic closure of the pulmonic valve in pulmonary hypertension.

Takahama H, McCully RB, Frantz RP, et al. Unraveling the RV ejection Doppler envelope: insight into pulmonary artery hemodynamics and disease severity. JACC Cardiovasc Imaging. 2017;10:1268–1277.

In pulmonary artery hypertension, this Doppler pattern appears to integrate indicators of pulmonary vascular load, and of right ventricular function. It also serves as a marker for adverse outcomes.

PISA

- Proximal isovelocity surface area (PISA): Flow converges on an orifice in layers of color Doppler, "candle flames," or isovelocities.
- Physics in action: PISA is an example of using color flow *aliasing* to perform calculations.

"A color Doppler hemisphere of blood flow multiplied by its velocity is divided by the flow velocity."

- PISA Formula:
  Surface area of flow hemisphere × aliasing velocity ÷ peak velocity.
- The flow rate through a hemispheric shell is equal to the flow rate through a mitral regurgitant orifice.
- $2\pi r^2 \times$ cm/s ÷ 5 m/s.
- Why 5 m/s? Mitral regurgitation is *assumed* to have this velocity.
- Why is πr^2 multiplied by 2? That is the formula for the surface area of a hemisphere.
- Caution in heart failure and in aortic stenosis, or dynamic left ventricular outflow obstruction:
  - Heart failure: Mitral regurgitation peak velocities may *drop* to 4 m/s or less.
  - Aortic stenosis or HOCM: Mitral regurgitation peak velocities may *rise* to 6 m/s or greater.
- Severe mitral regurgitation: effective regurgitant orifice area (ERO) >0.38 (rounded up to 0.4).
- PISA for mitral *stenosis* area requires angle correction.
- Misconception: The ultrasound machine prompts you to measure the integral of velocity (VTI) during the PISA calculation. This leads to confusion when trying to understand the formula.
  - The machine uses the *peak velocity* in the VTI tracing to calculate ERO, and it saves the VTI.
  - The VTI is then used to calculate *regurgitant volume* by multiplying the calculated ERO by this VTI.

THREE EASY PISAS

- "Eyeball" determination that mitral regurgitation is severe can be done by looking at the PISA radius.
- The purpose is to estimate the effective regurgitant orifice area (ERO).
- In the following three radius measurements, mitral regurgitation velocity has to be around 5 m/s for the math to be correct.

Rule 1: ERO = $r^2 \div 2$ (when aliasing velocity is set to 40 cm/s).

Rule 2 is the quick "eyeball" method:

- *Regurgitation is severe if PISA radius is 1 cm or greater.*
- Aliasing velocity has to be set to 30 cm/s.

Rule 3 works for any aliasing velocity:

- Regurgitation is severe if $1.9 \times r^2 \times$ aliasing velocity = 60 or greater (caution in prolapse).

MATHEMATICAL EXPLANATIONS

- $2\pi r^2$ is 6.28 in the numerator.
- Mitral regurgitation is in the denominator = 500 cm.
- Aliasing velocity is set to either 40 cm/s or 30 cm/s so that the numbers work out.
- The PISA radius in the formulas is manipulated so that ERO is 0.4 cm^2.

Mathematical Derivation of Rule 1:
$$[6.28 \times r^2 \times 40 \div 500] = [6.28 \times 40 \times r^2 \div 500] = [251 \times r^2 \div 500]$$
$$= [251 \div 500 \times r^2];$$
$$ERO = 1/2 \times r^2$$

Mathematical Derivation of Rule 2:
$$6.28 \times 30 \times 1^2 = 188.4$$
$$188.4 \div 500 = 0.38 \ ERO$$

If r is 1 cm or greater, ERO will be 0.38 or greater.

Mathematical Derivation of Rule 3:

- ERO × VTI = regurgitant volume.
- 6.28 gets divided by 3.25 to give the 1.9 in the formula.
- 3.25 comes from the reference below:
  - MR peak velocity is usually 3.25 times bigger than the MR VTI stroke distance.
  - The PISA radius is being used to correlate regurgitant volume with ERO.
- Caution: In mitral regurgitation due to mitral valve prolapse, PISA radius changes in size from early to late systole. The 1:3.25 relationship cannot be assumed (Fig. 3-3).
- Holosystolic mitral regurgitation is severe when $1.9 \times r^2 \times$ aliasing velocity = 60 or greater.
- Holosystolic mitral regurgitation is severe when regurgitant volume is 60 cc or greater.

Rossi A, Dujardin KS, Bailey KR, et al. Rapid estimation of regurgitant volume by the proximal isovelocity surface area method in mitral regurgitation: can continuous-wave Doppler echocardiography be omitted? J Am Soc Echocardiogr. 1998;11:138–148.

- *The mean ratio of maximal to integral of velocity (VTI) had a narrow range of variation (mean +/−SD, 3.25 +/−0.47).*
- *The estimated regurgitant volume, calculated as* **regurgitant flow ÷ 3.25***, showed an excellent correlation.*

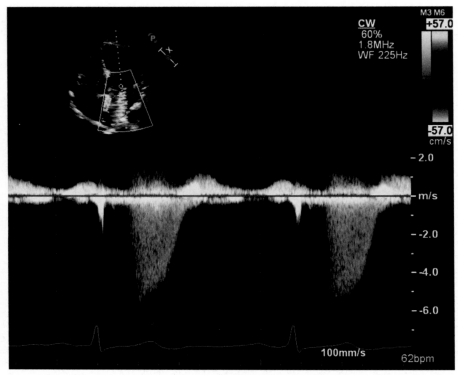

FIGURE 3-3. Mid to late systolic mitral regurgitation in mitral valve prolapse.

VENA CONTRACTA

- The narrowest portion of a regurgitant jet color flow signal.
- Simple measurement.
- No formula.
- Easily differentiates between mild and severe degrees of regurgitation.
- ≥0.7 cm is severe mitral regurgitation.

Roberts BJ, Grayburn PA. Color flow imaging of the vena contracta in mitral regurgitation: **technical considerations**. *J Am Soc Echocardiogr. 2003;16:1002–1006.*

TRICUSPID ANNULUS PEAK SYSTOLIC EXCURSION (TAPSE)

- Definition: A measure of longitudinal right ventricular function, defined as the distance of the systolic excursion of the right ventricular annulus along its longitudinal plane from an apical four-chamber view.
- Technique: Place an M-mode beam through the tricuspid annulus and measure the distance to peak systole (Fig. 3-4).
- Normal value: 17 mm or greater.
- Advantages: Simple, quick, reproducible.

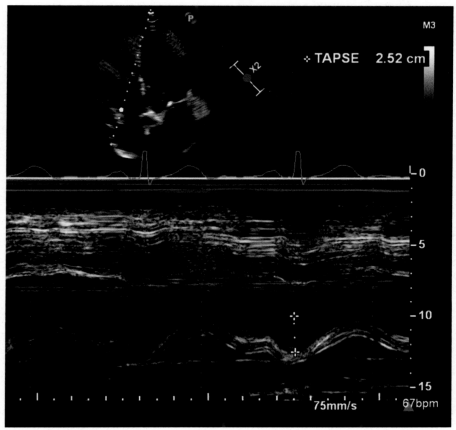

FIGURE 3-4. TAPSE.

- Disadvantages: Oversimplifies right ventricular function, angle dependent, affected by loading conditions.

S'TISSUE DOPPLER RIGHT VENTRICULAR SYSTOLIC EXCURSION VELOCITY

- This is a TAPSE equivalent.
- It measures longitudinal velocity of the tricuspid annulus, or the middle of the basal segment of the right ventricular free wall.
- Pulsed tissue Doppler velocities of <10 cm/s indicate abnormal right ventricular function.

NOTES

Echocardiographic Imaging

CHAPTER 4

2019 GUIDELINES

Mitchell C, Rahko PS, Blauwet LA, et al. Guidelines for performing a comprehensive transthoracic echocardiographic examination in adults: Recommendations from the American Society of Echocardiography. J Am Soc Echocardiogr. 2019;32:1–64.

- This comprehensive document is the **starting point** for learning and performing an echocardiographic examination in the adult.
- It is beautifully illustrated and comprehensive, and it includes an appendix with additional alternative views.
- Find and learn the highlighted key scanning points.
- Go to http://asecho.org to download the latest version.

STANDARD IMAGING

- The quality of echocardiographic images can vary widely from patient to patient.
- It is both operator and patient dependent.
- A standardized imaging approach is important to achieve study to study reproducibility.
- In order to obtain proper images, ultrasound must get around bone and lung tissue, and reach the heart.

Tajik AJ, Seward JB, Hagler DJ, et al. Two-dimensional real-time ultrasonic imaging of the heart and great vessels. Technique, image orientation, structure identification, and validation. Mayo Clin Proc. 1978;53:271–303.

PARASTERNAL LONG AXIS VIEW (PLAX)

- Parasternal images are best obtained with the patient in the left lateral decubitus position.

- Imaging advantages of the lateral decubitus position:
  - The heart moves away from under the sternum.
  - The rib interspaces separate more.
  - An ultrasound pathway around lung tissue becomes available.
  - The long axis view is parallel to the long axis of the heart.
- The major cardiac structures (possible abnormal findings in parentheses) in this view are:
  - The proximal ascending aorta, and a peephole view of the descending aorta behind the heart (aneurysm, dissection flap, atherosclerotic plaque).
  - The aortic valve (bicuspid valve, aortic valve endocarditis, calcification or thickening).
  - The left atrium (dilatation, sphericity, elongation, systolic expansion, myxomas).
  - The mitral valve, chordae, and papillary tips (prolapse, systolic anterior motion, rheumatic doming, endocarditis, annular calcification).
  - The basal and mid-left ventricular septum and inferolateral wall (basal septal hypertrophy, wall motion abnormalities).
  - Pericardium and pericardial space (effusion, pleuro/pericardial thickening is only rarely measurable when there is fluid on both sides of the pericardium).
  - Coronary sinus (dilates when there is a left superior vena cava).

Reynolds T, Abate K, Abate J. "Rib-hooks," "pressure points," and "hugs": **technical hints** for improving two-dimensional echocardiographic imaging. J Am Soc Echocardiogr. 1993;6:312–318.

RIGHT VENTRICULAR FOCUSED VIEW

- The right ventricular focused apical four-chamber view is used to perform linear measurements of the right ventricle.
- Technique:
  - Transducer is pointed medially toward the tricuspid valve.
  - Left ventricular apex is kept in the same position.
  - Mitral annulus is moved over to the side.
  - Tricuspid annulus is moved toward the center of the image.
- Measurements:
  - Basal right ventricular cavity diameter (maximum short-axis length of the basal right ventricular cavity, in the mid portion of the basal segment).
  - Mid right ventricular cavity diameter (at the level of the *left* ventricular papillary muscle tips).
  - Right ventricular intracavitary length.

RIGHT VENTRICULAR WALL THICKNESS

- Measurement technique:
  - Use the subcostal window.
  - Use the end-diastolic frame at the ECG R wave.
  - Identify and exclude: epicardial fat, pericardial wall, right ventricular trabeculations.

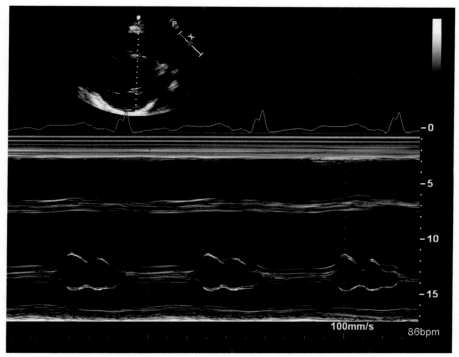

FIGURE 4-4. Delayed mitral valve closure (B bump). Dilated cardiomyopathy.

*Sahn DJ, DeMaria A, Kisslo J, et al. Recommendations regarding quantitation in **M-mode** echocardiography: results of a survey of echocardiographic measurements. Circulation. 1978;58:1072–1083.*

*Schiller NB, Shah PM, Crawford M, et al. Recommendations for quantitation of the **left ventricle** by two-dimensional echocardiography. J Am Soc Echocardiogr. 1989;2:358–367.*

STRAIN

- Measurement of myocardial motion (strain) and speed (strain rate).
- Either speckle tracking or (less often) tissue Doppler provide the measurement data.
- The calculations are displayed in multiple ways. This should not be allowed to create confusion.
- Global longitudinal strain (GLS) is revolutionizing the cardiac follow-up of certain cancer patients.
- Comparison with other techniques:
  - Cardiac motion in space is called *translation*.
  - Cardiac translation may affect perception of wall motion depending on the vantage point of the imaging transducer.
  - Strain is not affected in this way by transducer position because it uses adjacent areas of the heart for reference.
  - Strain complements calculation of left ventricular ejection fraction and analysis of regional wall motion.

Terminology

- Strain is the *change in length* between two points.
- In the left ventricle, strain can be the change in length between two points in the left ventricular wall.
- Normal systolic contraction of two points located on the long axis of the left ventricle can result in a 20% shorter distance between the two points.
- Negative global longitudinal strain of –20% (a 20% contraction and shortening, parallel to the long base to apex axis) can correspond to a normal left ventricular ejection fraction of 60%.
- Imaging pitfall: The inclusion of noncontracting pericardium in the points being analyzed by strain will give incorrect results.

Claus P, Omar AMS, Pedrizzeti G, et al. Tissue tracking technology for assessing cardiac mechanics: principles, **normal values**, and clinical applications. JACC Cardiovasc Imaging. 2015;8:1444–1460.

Collier P, Phelan D, Klein A. A test in context: myocardial strain measured by **speckle-tracking** echocardiography. J Am Coll Cardiol. 2017;69:1043–1056.

Knackstedt C, Bekkers SC, Schummers G, et al. **Fully automated** versus standard tracking of left ventricular ejection fraction and longitudinal strain: The FAST-EFs Multicenter Study. J Am Coll Cardiol. 2015;66:1456–1466.

Potter E, Marwick TH. Assessment of left ventricular function by echocardiography: the case for **routinely adding** global longitudinal strain to ejection fraction. JACC Cardiovasc Imaging. 2018;11:260–274.

Thavendiranathan P, Grant AD, Negishi T, et al. **Reproducibility** of echocardiographic techniques for sequential assessment of left ventricular ejection fraction and volumes: application to patients undergoing cancer chemotherapy. J Am Coll Cardiol. 2013;61:77–84.

Voigt JU, Pedrizzetti G, Lysyansky P, et al. Definitions for a **common standard** for 2D speckle tracking echocardiography: consensus document of the EACVI/ASE/Industry Task Force to standardize deformation imaging. J Am Soc Echocardiogr. 2015;28:183–193.

Yingchoncharoen T, Agarwal S, Popovic ZB, et al. **Normal ranges** of left ventricular strain: a meta-analysis. J Am Soc Echocardiogr. 2013;26:185–191.

CHAPTER 5

Diastology

GUIDELINES

Nagueh SF, Smiseth OA, Appleton CP, et al. Recommendations for the evaluation of left ventricular diastolic function by echocardiography. J Am Soc Echocardiogr. 2016;29:277–314.

- This is an essential document for the echocardiographer.
- There are various resources in the document that can be used without reading it from beginning to end.
- The pressure tracings, drawings, and echo images are easy to understand. They illustrate key concepts.
- Key points are separately highlighted and summarized in stepwise fashion.
- The tables and algorithms organize technical scanning information for the reader.

EVALUATION OF DIASTOLIC FUNCTION

- Left ventricular diastolic function can be evaluated by measuring indices of left ventricular:
  - Relaxation.
  - Restoring forces.
  - Diastolic compliance.
  - Filling pressure.
- By using a combination of indices, diastolic function can be graded and LV filling pressure estimated (Table 5-1).
- Diastolic function should be determined:
  - In unexplained exertional *dyspnea,* or other symptoms or signs of heart failure that cannot be attributed to reduced LV systolic function, or to diseases such as coronary artery disease, valve disease, pulmonary vascular disease, lung disease, or other diseases.

TABLE 5-1 • Grading of Diastolic Dysfunction

	Normal	Grade 1	Grade 2	Grade 3
LV relaxation	Normal	Impaired	Impaired	Impaired
LA pressure	Normal	Low or normal	Elevated	Elevated
Mitral E/A ratio	≥ 0.8	≤ 0.8	>0.8 to <2	>2
Average E/e' ratio	<10	<10	10–14	>14
Peak TR velocity (m/s)	<2.8	<2.8	>2.8	>2.8
LA volume index	Normal	Normal or increased	Increased	Increased

- To attempt to answer whether LV *filling pressure* is elevated in patients with heart failure and reduced LV ejection fraction, and when considering adjustment of diuretics or other heart failure medication.
- Grading of diastolic function can be used for *risk assessment* in asymptomatic subjects and in patients with heart disease.

Flachskampf FA, Biering-Sørensen T, Solomon SD, et al. Cardiac imaging to evaluate left ventricular diastolic function. JACC Cardiovasc Imaging. 2015;8:1071–1093.

Smiseth OA. Evaluation of left ventricular diastolic function: state of the art after 35 years with Doppler assessment. J Echocardiogr. 2018;16:55–64.

INDICATORS OF DIASTOLIC DYSFUNCTION

- E/e' ratio is seldom greater than 14 in individuals with normal filling pressures.
- Ar-A: An increase in pulmonary vein atrial reversal velocity duration versus mitral A duration is consistent with increased left ventricular end-diastolic pressure.
- A restrictive left ventricular filling pattern is found in dilated cardiomyopathy (Fig. 5-1).
- Left atrial size is increased (>34 mL/m²).
- Tricuspid regurgitation velocity is increased (>2.8 m/s).
- When systolic LV function is abnormal, diastolic function is presumed to be abnormal as well.
- In patients with clinical heart failure and apparently preserved systolic function, strain may demonstrate abnormal myocardial systolic and diastolic function.
- Caution when there is mitral annular calcium (MAC):
  - LV diastolic parameters, as measured by Doppler echocardiography, are altered in the presence of MAC.
  - This could be due to direct effects of MAC on annular function, or it might reflect truly reduced diastolic function.

Codolosa JN, Koshkelashvili N, Alnabelsi T, et al. **Effect** of mitral annular calcium on left ventricular diastolic parameters. Am J Cardiol. 2016;117:847–852.

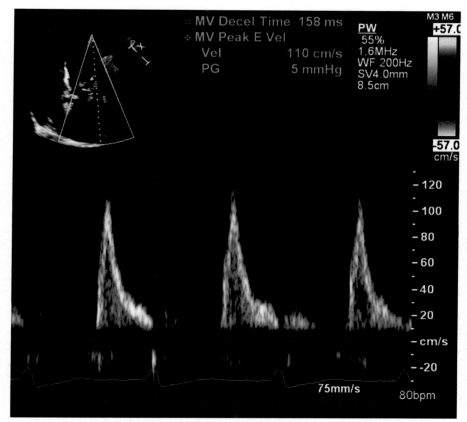

FIGURE 5-1. Restrictive left ventricular filling. Wall filter needs to be turned down.

Valsalva

- Imaging should be standardized by continuously recording mitral inflow using pulsed-wave Doppler for 10 seconds during the straining phase of the Valsalva maneuver.

- Response to Valsalva can help to distinguish normal diastolic LV filling from pseudonormal filling, and also to determine whether restrictive LV filling is reversible.

- A decrease during Valsalva in E/A ratio of ≥50% (not caused by E and A velocity fusion) is highly specific for increased LV filling pressures, and it supports the presence of diastolic dysfunction.

MITRAL INFLOW PATTERN AT THE LEAFLET TIPS

- Color flow is used to guide the placement of pulsed-wave Doppler sampling at the actual leaflet tips.

- Wall filters need adjustment so that the Doppler signal is not filtered out at the baseline, and duration measurements can be made.

- The duration of the A wave can be measured more easily by moving the pulsed-wave sample volume 5 mm closer to the mitral annulus.

- Left atrial size:
  - The left atrium increases in size in response to pressure and/or volume overload.
  - A normal left atrium becomes slightly larger in systole.
  - Systolic expansion of the left atrium may be visually perceptible in some patients.
  - Left atrial volumes should be measured at end systole when the left atrial chamber volume is largest.
  - The *geometry* of the left atrium may range from oval to spherical.
  - During imaging, the transducer should be carefully adjusted to maximize the size of the left atrial chamber dimensions.

DIASTOLIC PULMONARY VEIN FLOW

- When pulmonary vein flow enters the left atrium preferentially in diastole, the mitral valve is open and pulmonary vein pressure exceeds left atrial pressure, which in turn exceeds left ventricular pressure (Fig. 5-2).
- Normal pulmonary vein flow is preferentially *systolic* when left atrial pressure is normal.
- Systolic pulmonary vein inflow is generated by *suction*.
- Left atrial relaxation is responsible for the first systolic component.
- Subsequent systolic pulmonary venous inflow is created by apical displacement of the mitral annulus.

*Klein AL, Tajik AJ. Doppler assessment of **pulmonary venous flow** in healthy subjects and in patients with heart disease. J Am Soc Echocardiogr. 1991;4:379–392.*

RANGE AMBIGUITY WHEN SAMPLING PULMONARY VEIN FLOW

- When using pulsed wave Doppler in the apical views to interrogate the right pulmonary veins, the ultrasound computer may automatically switch to high pulse repetition frequency (HPRF) Doppler.

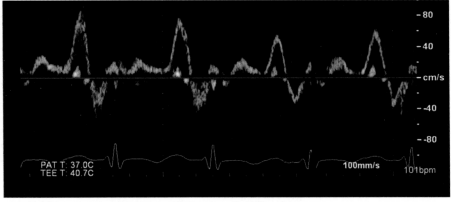

FIGURE 5-2. Diastolic dominant pulmonary vein inflow pattern.

- This creates range ambiguity.
- The pulmonary vein tracing may be *overlapped* by mitral Doppler flow signals.

ISOVOLUMIC RELAXATION TIME

- IVRT is the time from aortic valve closure to mitral valve opening.
- Prolongation of the IVRT indicates impaired left ventricular relaxation.
- Short IVRT indicates elevated left atrial pressure.
- Measurement technique:
  - Sample volume is obtained in the "five chamber view."
  - Sweep speed is maximized.
  - Sample volume is adjusted until both aortic valve closure spikes and mitral opening spikes are simultaneously recorded.

Oh JK, Tajik J. *The return of cardiac time intervals: the phoenix is rising. J Am Coll Cardiol. 2003;42:1471–1474.*

MYOCARDIAL PERFORMANCE INDEX

"Isovolumic contraction time plus isovolumic relaxation time divided by ejection time."

- The Tei index is also known as the myocardial performance index (MPI). The Doppler-derived MPI is a measure of combined systolic and diastolic myocardial performance.
- It is clinically useful in heart failure and in coronary artery disease.
- It is also calculated in the right heart by measuring the duration of tricuspid regurgitation and right ventricular outflow ejection time. Alternatively, it can be calculated by using pulsed-wave tissue Doppler.

Bruch C, Schmermund A, Marin D, et al. Tei-index in patients with mild-to-moderate congestive **heart failure**. Eur Heart J. 2000;21:1888–1895.

Kato M, Dote K, Sasaki S, et al. Myocardial performance index for assessment of left ventricular outcome in successfully recanalised anterior myocardial **infarction**. Heart. 2005;91:583–588.

Ogihara Y, Yamada N, Dohi K, et al. Utility of **right ventricular** Tei-index for assessing disease severity and determining response to treatment in patients with pulmonary arterial hypertension. J Cardiol. 2014;63:149–153.

HEPATIC VEINS

- Pulsed-wave interrogation is performed in the subcostal short-axis view.
- Sampling is done parallel to hepatic vein flow.
- Sample volume gate should be maximized.
- Sample volume is then adjusted to obtain a systolic and a diastolic wave, and an atrial reversal wave.
- Progressive increase in right ventricular filling pressures will:
  - Decrease the systolic filling velocity.
  - Cause diastolic velocities to increase and dominate the forward flow pattern.
  - Cause systolic and diastolic flow reversals to become evident.

- Diastolic flow reversals are found in pulmonary hypertension.
- Diastolic flow reversals that increase during expiration are found in pericardial constriction.
- Early-systolic flow reversals are found in right ventricular dysfunction.
- Late-systolic flow reversals are found in severe tricuspid regurgitation.

INTRACAVITARY GRADIENTS—VELOCITY OF PROPAGATION

- Flow moves forward in the left ventricle in diastole because there is an intracavitary gradient.
- It is possible to further analyze this gradient by measuring velocity of propagation.
- By analyzing the left ventricle one can make predictions:
  - A *dilated diffusely hypokinetic* left ventricle is predicted to have a restrictive filling pattern at the mitral valve leaflet tips because of a high gradient between the left atrium and the left ventricle in early diastole right after mitral leaflet opening.
  - Furthermore, downstream in this left ventricle, the flow moves forward at a slow velocity.
  - Conversely, a *small hypertrophied* left ventricle with normal systolic function will have a completely different mitral inflow pattern. In this ventricle, velocity of propagation may be increased because of a high intracavitary gradient.

MEASURING FLOW PROPAGATION VELOCITY

- Color M-mode provides Doppler information (which way, how fast) along the entire path of the M-mode beam.
- When the mitral valve opens in early diastole, flow accelerates toward the left ventricular apex.
- Placing the M-mode beam along the path of early diastolic mitral inflow provides spatial Doppler information about left ventricular intracavitary pressure gradients, and about left ventricular diastolic function.
- Measurement:
  - The slope of the propagation velocity is calculated as a line from the mitral annulus into the left ventricle.
  - The line follows the valve to apex contour of the color flow pattern, coinciding in time with the E wave.
  - The distance traveled, divided by how long it takes, is reported in cm/s.
  - The steeper the slope (fast blood propagation), the better the diastolic relaxation.
  - A slow velocity of propagation (<50 cm/s) indicates diastolic dysfunction.
  - The slow velocity is very obvious in many patients with dilated cardiomyopathy. In these patients, pulsed-wave Doppler at the mitral leaflet tips shows rapid early diastolic acceleration and deceleration.
  - If the pulsed Doppler E velocity is more than 1.4 times the velocity of propagation, left atrial pressure is increased.

TABLE 5-2 • Atrial Fibrillation: Parameters of Abnormal Diastolic Function

Deceleration time (ms)	≤160
E acceleration (cm/s²)	≥1900
IVRT (ms)	≤65
PVEIN DT* (ms)	≤220
E/velocity of propagation ratio	>1.4
E/e' ratio	≥11

Deceleration time of pulmonary vein diastolic velocity.

- Pitfall: Hypertrophic and restrictive cardiomyopathies with diastolic dysfunction may appear to have rapid velocities of propagation because of left ventricular intracavitary flow that takes place *before* the actual early filling of interest.

Chirillo F, Brunazzi MC, Barbiero M, et al. Estimating mean pulmonary wedge pressure in patients with chronic **atrial fibrillation** from transthoracic Doppler indexes of mitral and pulmonary venous flow velocity. J Am Coll Cardiol. 1997;30:19–26.

Maniu CV, Nishimura RA, Tajik AJ. Tachycardia during the Valsalva maneuver: a sign of normal diastolic filling pressures. J Am Soc Echocardiogr. 2004;17:634–637.

Nagueh SF, Kopelen HA, Quinones MA. Assessment of left ventricular filling pressures by Doppler in the presence of **atrial fibrillation**. Circulation. 1996;94:2138–2145. (See Table 5-2.)

Temporelli PL, Scapellato F, Corra U, et al. Estimation of pulmonary wedge pressure by transmitral Doppler in patients with chronic heart failure and **atrial fibrillation**. Am J Cardiol. 1999;83:724–727.

NOTES

Heart Failure

HEART TRANSPLANTATION

- The biatrial surgical transplant technique (Fig. 6-1) is being replaced by the bicaval technique: superior and inferior cava anastomosis with left atrial excision to the base of the left atrial appendage.
- Advantages:
  - Right atrial size remains small.
  - There is less tricuspid regurgitation.

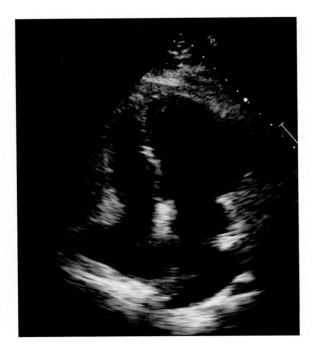

FIGURE 6-1. The atrial suture line can be demonstrated on the echo of some heart transplant patients.

- Less likelihood of need for a post-op pacemaker.
- Atrial filling pressures tend to remain normal.
- Stress echo can help with pretransplant donor heart selection.
- Following transplantation:
  - Right ventricular: TAPSE, S', strain, and fractional area change can remain lower than normal.
  - 3D echo can be used to guide myocardial biopsy while imaging the tricuspid valve.

Badano LP, Miglioranza MH, Edvardsen T, et al. Recommendations for the use of cardiac imaging to assess and follow patients after heart transplantation. Eur Heart J Cardiovasc Imaging. 2015;16:919–948.

Bhatia SJ, Kirshenbaum JM, Shemin RJ, et al. Time course of resolution of pulmonary hypertension and right ventricular remodeling after orthotopic cardiac transplantation. Circulation. 1987;76:819–826.

Costanzo MR, Dipchand A, Starling R, et al. The International Society of Heart and Lung Transplantation **Guidelines** for the care of heart transplant recipients. J Heart Lung Transplant. 2010;29:914–956.

Ingvarsson A, Werther Evaldsson A, Waktare J, et al. Normal reference ranges for transthoracic echocardiography following heart transplantation. J Am Soc Echocardiogr. 2018;31:349–360.

Jacob S, Sellke F. Is **bicaval** orthotopic heart transplantation superior to the biatrial technique? Interact Cardiovasc Thorac Surg. 2009;9:333–342.

Leone O, Gherardi S, Targa L, et al. Stress echocardiography as a **gatekeeper to donation** in aged marginal donor hearts: anatomic and pathologic correlations of abnormal stress echocardiography results. J Heart Lung Transplant. 2009;28:1141–1149.

Nguyen V, Cantarovich M, Cecere R, et al. Tricuspid regurgitation after cardiac transplantation: how many **biopsies** are too many? J Heart Lung Transplant. 2005;24:S227–S231.

*Platts D, Brown M, Javorsky G, et al. Comparison of fluoroscopic versus real-time three-dimensional transthoracic **echocardiographic guidance** of endomyocardial biopsies. Eur J Echocardiogr. 2010;11:637–643.*

PERICARDIAL EFFUSION FOLLOWING HEART TRANSPLANTATION

- Predictors of effusion formation after heart transplant:
  - Weight difference between recipient and donor (recipient weight > donor weight)—small donor heart.
  - Lack of a previous median sternotomy.
- Cardiac perforation is a possible cause of an effusion following myocardial biopsy.
- Late-onset, persistent, or increasing pericardial effusions in a transplant patient should raise concerns about transplant rejection.
- Purulent pericarditis should be a consideration, given the altered immune status.

Canver CC, Patel AK, Kosolcharoen P, et al. Fungal purulent constrictive pericarditis in a heart transplant patient. Ann Thorac Surg. 1998;65:1792–1794.

Hauptman PJ, Couper GS, Aranki SF, et al. Pericardial effusions after cardiac transplantation. J Am Coll Cardiol. 1994;23:1625–1629.

Valantine HA, Hunt SA, Gibbons R, et al. Increasing pericardial effusion in cardiac transplant recipients. Circulation. 1989;79:603–609.

DIASTOLIC FILLING IN HEART TRANSPLANT PATIENTS

- A restrictive filling pattern is common in transplant patients. Explanation: Donor hearts are usually obtained from healthy young individuals with preserved diastolic suction.
- Tricuspid regurgitation velocity can be used as a surrogate for mean left atrial pressure.
- No single diastolic parameter appears reliable enough to predict graft rejection.

*Dumesnil JG, Gaudreault G, Honos GN, et al. Use of **Valsalva** maneuver to unmask left ventricular diastolic function abnormalities by Doppler echocardiography in patients with coronary artery disease or systemic hypertension. Am J Cardiol. 1991;68:515–519.*

*Garcia MJ, Ares MA, Asher C, et al. An index of early left ventricular filling that combined with pulsed Doppler peak E velocity may estimate **capillary wedge pressure**. J Am Coll Cardiol. 1997;29:448–454.*

*Lam CS, Han L, Ha JW, et al. The mitral **L wave**: a marker of pseudonormal filling and predictor of heart failure in patients with left ventricular hypertrophy. J Am Soc Echocardiogr. 2005;18:336–341.*

*Nagueh SF, Middleton KJ, Kopelen HA, et al. **Doppler tissue** imaging: a noninvasive technique for evaluation of left ventricular relaxation and estimation of filling pressures. J Am Coll Cardiol. 1997;30:1527–1533.*

*Ommen SR, Nishimura RA, Appleton CP, et al. Clinical utility of Doppler echocardiography and tissue Doppler imaging in the estimation of left ventricular **filling pressures**: a comparative simultaneous Doppler-catheterization study. Circulation. 2000;102:1788–1794.*

*Paulus WJ, Tschöpe C, Sanderson JE, et al. **How to diagnose** diastolic heart failure: a consensus statement on the diagnosis of heart failure with normal left ventricular ejection fraction by the Heart Failure and Echocardiography Associations of the European Society of Cardiology. Eur Heart J. 2007;28:2539–2550.*

*Pinamonti B, Di Lenarda A, Sinagra G, et al. Restrictive left ventricular **filling pattern** in dilated cardiomyopathy assessed by Doppler echocardiography: clinical, echocardiographic and hemodynamic correlations and prognostic implications. Heart Muscle Disease Study Group. J Am Coll Cardiol. 1993;22:808–815.*

*Rossvoll O, Hatle LK. **Pulmonary venous** flow velocities recorded by transthoracic Doppler ultrasound: relation to left ventricular diastolic pressures. J Am Coll Cardiol. 1993;21:1687–1696.*

*Sagie A, Benjamin EJ, Galderisi M, et al. **Reference values** for Doppler indexes of left ventricular diastolic filling in the elderly. J Am Soc Echocardiogr. 1993;6:570–576.*

Santos M, Rivero J, McCullough SD, et al. E/e' ratio in patients with unexplained dyspnea: lack of accuracy in estimating left ventricular filling pressure. Circ Heart Fail. 2015;8:749–756.

*Sohn DW, Chai IH, Lee DJ, et al. Assessment of **mitral annulus** velocity by Doppler tissue imaging in the evaluation of left ventricular diastolic function. J Am Coll Cardiol. 1997;30:474–480.*

LVAD FOR HEART FAILURE

- An echocardiographic study of an LVAD patient should start by confirming that there is a cannula pulling blood from the LV apex to the pump, and that the outgoing pump cannula delivers the blood into the ascending aorta.
- Pump differential pressure: Difference between aortic pressure and left ventricular pressure.
- Affected by:
  - Pump speed.
  - Systolic blood pressure.
  - Left ventricular pressure.
  - Existing reserve of native left ventricular contractility.
  - Cannula flow.
  - Cannula obstruction.
  - Cannula twisting or pinching.
- Role of echo: Aortic valve opening is used along with pump parameters to analyze how much blood goes through the aortic valve in relation to flow through the apical cannula (Fig. 6-2).
- Examples:
  - When the pump is set to *low speeds*, more flow is expected through the aortic valve. This indicates the presence of some residual myocardial contractility.
  - When the pump is set to *high speeds*, the myocardium is being rested. Flow goes to the apical cannula. Echo shows little or no flow through the aortic valve in systole.
- Echocardiographic findings after LVAD insertion:
  - Left ventricular chamber dimensions are expected to decrease.
  - Apical tethering of the mitral leaflets is expected to decrease.
  - The position of the interatrial septum is expected to change when left atrial pressures get lower. The position and curvature of the thin membrane of the fossa ovalis is a "barometer" of the pressure differences between the atria.
  - Mitral inflow pattern is expected to reflect lower left atrial and lower left ventricular pressures.

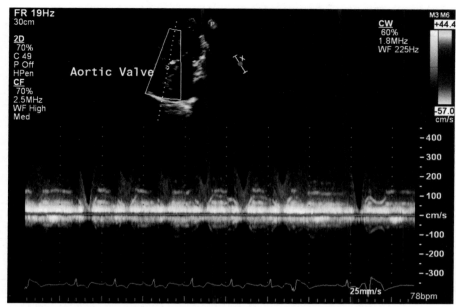

FIGURE 6-2. Ventricular assist device. Continuous systolic and diastolic aortic regurgitation.

- Examples of favorable changes in mitral inflow:
  - Lower E velocity.
  - Longer early diastolic deceleration time.
- Echo findings that suggest LVAD cannula obstruction:
  - Left-to-right displacement of the interventricular septum.
  - Left-to-right displacement of the interatrial septum.
  - Worsening mitral regurgitation.
  - Increase in systolic aortic leaflet excursion.
  - Change of the color flow at the cannula.

Lam KM, Ennis S, O'Driscoll G, et al. Observations from non-invasive measures of **right heart** hemodynamics in left ventricular assist device patients. J Am Soc Echocardiogr. 2009;22:1055–1062.

Topilsky Y, Hasin T, McGregor CG, et al. **Mitral** valve regurgitation in patients supported on continuous flow pumps. Echocardiography. 2011;28:E202–E204.

Topilsky Y, Hasin T, Oh JK, et al. Echocardiographic variables after left ventricular assist device implantation associated with adverse outcome. Circ Cardiovasc Imaging. 2011;4:648–661.

Topilsky Y, Oh JK, Atchison FW, et al. Echocardiographic findings in stable outpatients with properly functioning **HeartMate** II left ventricular assist devices. J Am Soc Echocardiogr. 2011;24:157–169.

Vollkron M, Voitl P, Ta J, et al. **Suction events** during left ventricular support and ventricular arrhythmias. J Heart Lung Transplant. 2007;26:819–825.

- Mortality and heart failure after LVAD surgery are related to echocardiographic evidence of:
  - Inefficient unloading of the left ventricle.

- Persistence of right ventricular dysfunction.
- Increased estimated LA pressure.
- Short ratio of mitral deceleration time to E-wave velocity.
- Leftward deviation of the interventricular septum.

CARDIAC RESYNCHRONIZATION THERAPY IN HEART FAILURE

- Echocardiographic measurements:
  - M-mode septal to posterior wall motion delay >130 ms.
  - Tissue Doppler time difference to peak velocity between the anteroseptal and posterolateral walls.
  - Speckle tracking radial strain.
  - 3D systolic dyssynchrony index: standard deviation of the time taken to reach minimum regional volume for myocardial segments.
  - Pulsed-wave Doppler interventricular delay: delay between onset of right ventricular and left ventricular outflow ejection.

Gorcsan J 3rd, Abraham T, Agler DA, et al. Echocardiography for cardiac resynchronization therapy: recommendations for performance and reporting. J Am Soc Echocardiogr. 2008;21:191–213.
This document contains extensive illustrations of the dyssynchrony measurements listed above.

Kapetanakis S, Bhan A, Murgatroyd F, et al. Real-time 3D echo in patient selection for cardiac resynchronization therapy. JACC Cardiovasc Imaging. 2011;4:16–26.

Lim P, Buakhamsri A, Popovic ZB, et al. Longitudinal strain delay index by speckle tracking imaging: a new marker of response to cardiac resynchronization therapy. Circulation. 2008;118:1130–1137.

VIDEOS

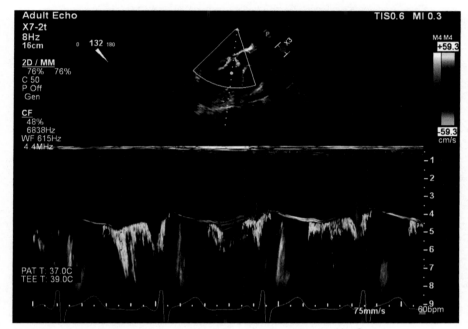

FIGURE 6-3. Aortic regurgitation impinging on the anterior mitral leaflet.

- **Quiz: Can you find the systolic flow propagation?**
  Hint: Bright systolic yellow line, third cardiac cycle, distance over time.

VIDEO 6-1. Visual timing of color flow: *Systolic* mitral and tricuspid regurgitation. *Diastolic* aortic regurgitation. *Systolic and diastolic* caval inflow.

VIDEO 6-2. Global longitudinal strain.

VIDEO 6-3. Strain in atrial fibrillation.

VIDEOS 6-4 (A-C). Diastolic dominant pulmonary vein inflow.

VIDEO 6-5. Atrial fibrillation. Elevated left atrial pressure.

VIDEO 6-6. Color flow artifact: The color extends past the anatomic descending aorta.

VIDEO 6-7. Mirror color flow artifact.

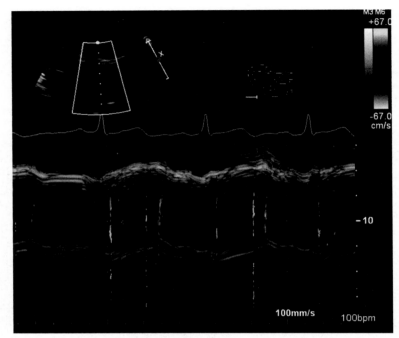

FIGURE 6-4. Filter saturation artifacts.

VIDEO 6-8. Closed aortic valve. Ventricular assist device.

VIDEO 6-9. Apical left ventricular cannula. Ventricular assist device.

VIDEO 6-10. Isovolumic relaxation time.

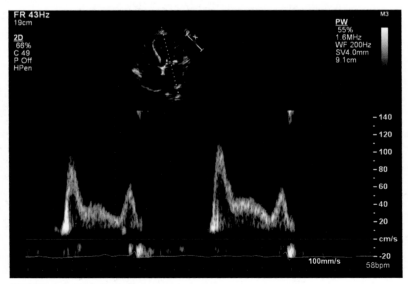

FIGURE 6-5. Mid-diastolic L wave.

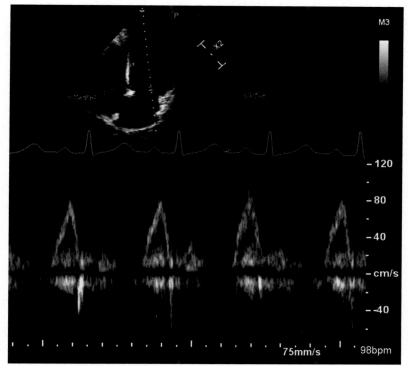

FIGURE 6-6. Mitral inflow: E-wave and A-wave fusion.

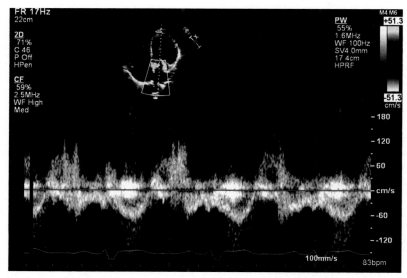

FIGURE 6-7. Range ambiguity during pulmonary vein HPRF Doppler imaging. Systolic mitral regurgitation signal superimposed on pulmonary vein inflow.

NOTES

CHAPTER 7

Coronary Artery Disease

The "bread and butter" of adult cardiology is coronary artery disease.

INTRODUCTION

"Look locally—interpret globally."

- Regional left ventricular wall motion analysis is the cornerstone of echocardiographic imaging in coronary artery disease.
- Regional left ventricular wall motion abnormalities are indicators of myocardial ischemia during a stress test.
- Regional left ventricular wall motion abnormalities are present in acute myocardial infarction.
- In addition to localizing myocardial infarction, echocardiography serves to diagnose *complications* of infarction.
- Anterior myocardial infarction can be complicated by an apical left ventricular aneurysm.
- Inferior myocardial infarction can be complicated by mitral regurgitation.
- Pulmonary edema and a new murmur, in a patient with myocardial infarction, may indicate either papillary muscle rupture or ventricular septal rupture. Echocardiography helps to identify these critical complications.
- Right ventricular infarction is an important complication of inferior myocardial infarction, and echocardiography is used for diagnosis and subsequent management.
- The electrocardiogram is utilized in conjunction with the echocardiogram in *all* patients with coronary artery disease.
- Basic roles of echocardiography:
  - Regional left ventricular wall motion analysis.
  - Stress testing for myocardial ischemia.
  - Complications of myocardial infarction.
  - Differential diagnosis of chest pain.

ROLE OF ECHO IN ACUTE MYOCARDIAL INFARCTION

- The decision for initiating treatment in acute ST-elevation myocardial infarction is made quickly and is based on the ECG and cardiac symptoms.
- The echocardiogram serves to help exclude alternative diagnoses for the cause of chest pain, such as aortic dissection or pericarditis.
- The echocardiogram can help diagnose the following *complications* of myocardial infarction:
    - Apical left ventricular aneurysm in anterior myocardial infarction.
    - Apical left ventricular thrombus.
    - Basal inferior aneurysm.
    - Mitral regurgitation and/or papillary muscle rupture.
    - Ventricular septal rupture.
    - Left ventricular pseudoaneurysm (ventricular rupture into the pericardial space).
    - Right ventricular infarction.

*Marangelli V, Cacciavillani L, Pontarollo S, et al. Images in cardiovascular medicine. Three-dimensional imaging in **rupture of papillary muscle** after acute myocardial infarction. Circulation. 2005;111:e385–e387.*

LOCALIZED REGIONAL VS DIFFUSE ST-SEGMENT ABNORMALITIES

- The role of echocardiography in coronary artery disease centers on *regional* wall motion analysis of the left ventricle.
- The ECG of myocardial infarction is complemented by regional left ventricular wall motion on echo to help *localize* and to *define extent* of infarction.
- Both the ECG and the echocardiogram serve to localize the affected territory in coronary artery disease.
- In contrast, the ECGs of pericarditis and myocarditis show *diffuse* ST-segment abnormalities.
- The echocardiogram helps to distinguish between myocarditis and pericarditis.
- There should be diffuse left ventricular motion abnormalities, as well as left ventricular cavity dilatation, on the echocardiogram of patients with myocarditis.
- There should be a pericardial effusion on the echocardiogram of patients with pericarditis.
- Caution: Pericarditis and myocarditis are not always mutually exclusive. Elevated troponins in pericarditis may indicate coexisting myocarditis.

*Wang K, Asinger RW, Marriott HJ. **ST-segment elevation** in conditions other than acute myocardial infarction. N Engl J Med. 2003;349:2128–2135.*

DIFFERENTIAL DIAGNOSIS OF CHEST PAIN

- Clinical importance of echo in patients with chest pain and suspected coronary artery disorders (angina, acute myocardial infarction): Echo findings may uncover an *alternative* explanation for chest pain.
- Pericarditis (pericardial fluid is present, wall motion abnormalities are absent).

- Aortic dissection (aortic regurgitation, pericardial effusion, dissection flap).
- Myocarditis (diffuse rather than localized wall motion abnormalities on echo, and diffuse rather than localizing ECG changes, elevated cardiac enzymes).

WALL MOTION ANALYSIS OF THE LAD ARTERY TERRITORY

- The left anterior descending artery wraps around the left ventricular apex. The most distal and therefore the most vulnerable territory can be the apical inferior wall.
- In the apical two-chamber view, it is possible to determine whether the wall motion abnormality at the apical inferior wall is due to right coronary or left coronary disease.

PITFALLS OF REGIONAL WALL MOTION ANALYSIS

- Regional left ventricular wall motion abnormalities are usually reliable indicators of coronary artery disease.
- However, the echocardiogram of a normal person may sometimes show a regional wall motion abnormality such as can be seen following inferior myocardial infarction.
- Of all the left ventricular walls, the *basal inferior wall* is the most prone to erroneous interpretation. Echocardiography is considered highly specific (rarely wrong when abnormal) for the diagnosis of myocardial ischemia. The basal inferior wall can be an exception to this rule (Fig. 7-3).
- This is particularly evident in patients with left ventricular hypertrophy. The hypertrophy may spare the basal inferior left ventricular wall, and the relatively thin basal inferior wall may simulate a prior inferior myocardial infarction.
- Prominent "septal" Q waves on the ECG (due to the hypertrophy) may further confound the clinical picture by suggesting the presence of myocardial infarction when there are no regional left ventricular wall motion abnormalities on echo.
- The basal inferior septum retains its *normal* thickness and motion in the *normal* patient.
- The apical lateral left ventricular wall will not be falsely abnormal but may often be difficult to image. Contrast enhancement will help.
- The apical cap is analyzed for motion, rather than for presence or absence of thickening.
- It will *not* be falsely abnormal.

APICAL LEFT VENTRICULAR ANEURYSM

- Anterior myocardial infarction can be complicated by an apical left ventricular aneurysm.
- Echocardiography can detect some but not all of the consequences of a left ventricular aneurysm.
- Apical left ventricular thrombus is one such consequence. The thrombus "seals" the aneurysm, but thromboembolism may occur.

- The other two clinical consequences are left heart failure and ventricular arrhythmias.
- It is a misconception that an apical left ventricular aneurysm is complicated by rupture.
- A "ruptured aneurysm" is actually called a pseudoaneurysm.
  - This is a distinct entity with a different natural history.
  - It requires urgent surgical intervention.
- A pseudoaneurysm does not evolve from a true aneurysm.
  - An aneurysm is a bulge. A pseudoaneurysm is a hole.
  - Aneurysm has only three complications: thromboembolism, arrhythmias, and systolic left ventricular dysfunction (manifested as heart failure).
- Imaging tip for apical aneurysms: Make your own acoustic standoff:
  - An aneurysm may be too close to the transducer in some patients.
  - Aside from using contrast ventriculography, an acoustic standoff can be made by *overfilling an intravenous solution bag* so that it is stretched and free of air bubbles.
  - Some of the near-field artifacts that make the echocardiographic examination of an apical aneurysm difficult will be removed by interposing the fluid filled bag between the transducer and the skin.
  - Harmonic imaging dramatically reduces ultrasound artifacts due to the standoff.

Tallarico D, Chiavari PA, Mollo P, et al. *Images in cardiovascular medicine. Left ventricular **pseudoaneurysm**: echocardiographic and intraoperative images. Circulation. 2005;111:e35–e36.*

APICAL LEFT VENTRICULAR THROMBUS

- Thrombus develops in areas of akinesis where there is nonviable myocardium. It has a predilection for the left ventricular apex.
- Thrombus may develop as early as a few hours after onset of infarction with a peak incidence at 3 days. It can occur even later after myocardial infarction, if apical wall motion does not improve.
- The most important complication of thrombus is the possibility of an embolism and consequent stroke.
- The likelihood of embolism is highest in the first 2 weeks after acute MI, and it decreases over the next 6 weeks. After that, the thrombus becomes adherent to the wall with endothelialization, and the likelihood of embolism decreases.
- Thrombus mobility is an ominous echocardiographic finding.
- A pedunculated (narrow base of attachment) independently mobile thrombus has a higher chance of embolizing than a laminated sessile thrombus with a broad base.
- Over time, the appearance may go back and forth between a mural and a protruding thrombus.
- The echocardiographic appearance of a thrombus is that of a mass (Fig. 7-1).

- The fact that there is an underlying wall motion abnormality separates it from other possibilities such as a tumor or an artifact. The apical location makes endocarditis highly unlikely.
- The underlying wall motion abnormality, combined with a mass (that may or may not protrude into the cavity) is the echocardiographic hallmark of a thrombus.
- It must be distinguished from other findings such as a false tendon or abnormally trabeculated myocardium. The latter is especially common in patients with left ventricular hypertrophy or noncompaction.

SCANNING TIPS

- Contrast should be used if needed.
- Harmonics should be turned off, and on again, to see what gives better detail.
- The transducer focus should be adjusted.
- An *acoustic standoff* between the transducer and the patient can be useful.
- A higher-frequency transducer is better for imaging the left ventricular apex. The resolution is higher, and the dead zone is shorter.
- The *dead zone* is the region closest to the transducer where ultrasound reflections do not depict anatomy accurately.

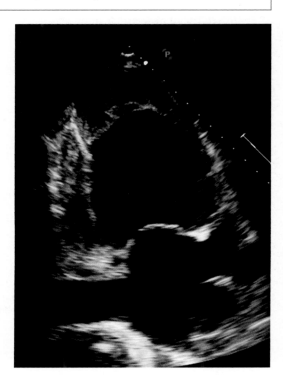

FIGURE 7-1. Apical left ventricular aneurysm. Superimposed mural apical left ventricular thrombus. No evident left atrial appendage thrombus.

- Causes of the dead zone:
  - Insufficient distance/time for the transducer to switch from transmitting to receiving.
  - Lack of a consolidated reflective wave of ultrasound at this short distance from the transducer.

Delewi R, Zijlstra F, Piek JJ. Left ventricular thrombus **formation** *after acute myocardial infarction. Heart. 2012;98: 1743–1749.*

Gianstefani S, Douiri A, Delithanasis I, et al. Incidence and predictors of early left **ventricular thrombus** *after ST-elevation myocardial infarction in the contemporary era of primary percutaneous coronary intervention. Am J Cardiol. 2014;113: 1111–1116.*

Haugland JM, Asinger RW, Mikell FL, et al. **Embolic potential** *of left ventricular thrombi detected by two-dimensional echocardiography. Circulation. 1984;70:588–598.*

Thrombus mobility and protrusion can help in the identification of embolic potential.

CHEST PAIN IN THE EMERGENCY ROOM—ROLE OF ECHO

- Echo is useful in the assessment of patients with low-risk chest pain in the emergency department.
- Stress echo testing provides incremental value in chest pain evaluation.
- Echo can help anticipate possible future cardiac events.
- A normal stress echo in an ER patient suggests a low likelihood of future cardiac events.
- Increased use of myocardial strain analysis in the future is expected to help in the management of chronic coronary artery disease.

Aldous S, Richards AM, Cullen L, et al. The **incremental value** *of stress testing in patients with acute chest pain beyond serial cardiac troponin testing. Emerg Med J. 2016;33:319–324.*

Conti A, Sammicheli L, Gallini C, et al. Assessment of patients with low-risk chest pain in the emergency department: head-to-head **comparison** *of exercise stress echocardiography and exercise myocardial SPECT. Am Heart J. 2005;149: 894–901.*

Dahslett T, Karlsen S, Grenne B, et al. Early assessment of **strain** *echocardiography can accurately exclude significant coronary artery stenosis in suspected non-ST-segment elevation acute coronary syndrome. J Am Soc Echocardiogr. 2014;27:512–519.*

Fleischmann KE, Lee TH, Come PC, et al. Echocardiographic predictors of **complications** *in patients with chest pain. Am J Cardiol. 1997;79:292–298.*

Hickman M, Swinburn JM, Senior R. Wall thickening assessment with tissue **harmonic** *echocardiography results in improved risk stratification for patients with non-ST-segment elevation acute chest pain. Eur J Echocardiogr. 2004;5:142–148.*

Kontos MC, Arrowood JA, Paulsen WH, et al. Early echocardiography can predict **cardiac events** *in emergency department patients with chest pain. Ann Emerg Med. 1998;31:550–557.*

Rybicki FJ, Udelson JE, Peacock WF, et al. **Appropriate utilization** *of cardiovascular imaging in emergency department patients with chest pain. J Am Coll Cardiol. 2016;67:853–879.*

Sabia P, Abbott RD, Afrookteh A, et al. Importance of two-dimensional echocardiographic assessment of left ventricular **systolic function** *in patients presenting to the emergency room with cardiac-related symptoms. Circulation. 1991;84:1615– 1624.*

Savari SI, Haugaa KH, Zahid W, et al. Layer-specific quantification of myocardial deformation by **strain** *echocardiography may reveal significant coronary artery disease in patients with non-ST-segment elevation acute coronary syndrome. JACC Cardiovasc Imaging. 2013;6:535–544.*

WALL MOTION ON ECHO COMPARED WITH THE ECG

- The ECG hallmark of myocardial infarction is the Q wave.
- The ECG hallmark of myocardial *injury* is ST-segment elevation.
- The ECG hallmark of myocardial *ischemia* is ST-segment depression.
- Echocardiography can demonstrate the presence of myocardial ischemia during a stress test as a new left ventricular wall motion abnormality.
- Acute myocardial injury in a patient with chest pain and ST-segment elevation (in two contiguous leads) is treated emergently without waiting for an echocardiogram (or for cardiac enzyme results). The echocardiogram (when performed) will confirm the diagnosis by showing left ventricular wall motion abnormalities (Fig. 7-2).
- Aneurysm can complicate myocardial infarction. Electrocardiography makes the diagnosis after the fact; the ECG sign of aneurysm is *persistent* (more than 30 days) ST-segment elevation. The echocardiogram can *readily* demonstrate the aneurysm.
- Patients with myocardial enzyme elevations indicating myocardial infarction do not always develop regional echocardiographic wall motion abnormalities. Usually this denotes a small infarct. Absence of regional wall motion abnormalities under these circumstances is typically associated with a better prognosis.

Dubnow MH, Burchell HB, Titus JL. Postinfarction ventricular aneurysm. A clinicomorphologic and electrocardiographic study of 80 cases. Am Heart J. 1965;70:753–760.

Utility of persistent ST-segment elevation for more than a month following myocardial infarction as an indicator of left ventricular aneurysm.

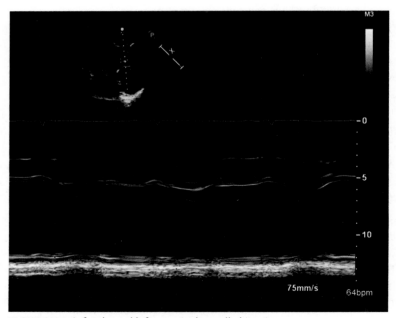

FIGURE 7-2. Inferolateral left ventricular wall akinesis.

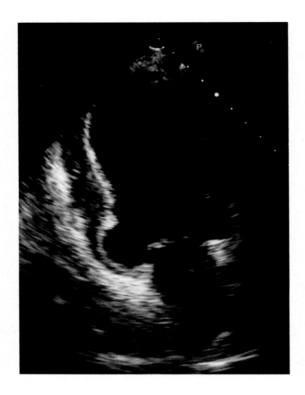

FIGURE 7-3. Basal inferior aneurysm.

RIGHT VENTRICULAR INFARCTION

- A complication of *inferior* myocardial infarction.
- Clinical clue: Q waves and ST elevation on the ECG in leads II, III, and AVF, combined with jugular venous distention.
- The right ventricle is a "volume" ventricle (rather than a "pressure" ventricle). It adapts to increased volume loads by temporarily increasing in size.
- Right heart failure in the absence of pulmonary hypertension:
  - Variable degrees of increased right ventricular *volume* may be evident on echo.
  - There may be paradoxical motion of the interventricular septum because of the volume overload.
  - Acute functional tricuspid regurgitation may develop due to tricuspid annular dilatation.
  - Tricuspid regurgitation velocities are characteristically low.
  - Tricuspid annular plane systolic excursion (TAPSE) is decreased, indicating decreased right ventricular longitudinal systolic function.
- Increased right atrial pressures:
  - Determined by examining the inferior vena cava: Increased cava diameter, loss or blunting of respiratory diameter changes.
  - Right atrial enlargement may not develop immediately.
  - There may be a tricuspid regurgitation late systolic cutoff due to rapidly rising right atrial pressures in a small non-adapted right atrium.

- Right-to-left atrial septal displacement may be seen.
- A preexisting foramen ovale may open up to depressurize the right atrium. Saline injection will show a *right-to-left* shunt.

Diagnosis and Treatment

- Echo determines relative amount of left ventricular inferior wall systolic dysfunction versus right ventricular systolic dysfunction and dilatation.
- Recognition and proper treatment with *fluids instead of diuretics* may be lifesaving.

Prognosis

- Recovery is expected, but lethal cardiogenic shock may occur in some patients.
- Occasionally, a survivor of an undiagnosed prior massive right ventricular infarction will present to the echo lab as right heart failure without pulmonary hypertension. The hypokinetic basal inferior left ventricular wall on echo, and the inferior infarct on ECG, help to confirm this diagnosis.

Park SJ, Park JH, Lee HS, et al. Impaired RV global longitudinal **strain** is associated with poor long-term clinical outcomes in patients with acute inferior STEMI. JACC Cardiovasc Imaging. 2015;8:161–169.

POSTINFARCTION LEFT VENTRICULAR OUTFLOW OBSTRUCTION

- Patients with acute anterior myocardial infarction may develop cardiogenic shock due to new onset of dynamic left ventricular outflow obstruction.
- There is usually a long-standing history of hypertension and a small body mass index.
- This is a rare but treatable cause of cardiogenic shock.
- On echo there are:
  - An apical left ventricular aneurysm.
  - Basal to midventricular septal hypertrophy (adjacent to the area of apical infarction).
  - Dynamic left ventricular outflow obstruction.

Chockalingam A, Tejwani L, Aggarwal K, et al. Dynamic left ventricular outflow tract obstruction in acute myocardial infarction with shock: cause, effect, and coincidence. Circulation. 2007;116:e110–e113.

Haley JH, Sinak LJ, Tajik AJ, et al. Dynamic left ventricular outflow tract obstruction in acute coronary syndromes: an important cause of **new systolic murmur** and cardiogenic shock. Mayo Clin Proc. 1999;74:901–906.

CORONARY ARTERY DISEASE (CAD) AND HEART FAILURE WITH REDUCED EJECTION FRACTION (HFrEF)

- Two most common causes of HFrEF: coronary artery disease and hypertension.
- Echocardiographic findings in HFrEF and CAD:
  - Left ventricular chamber enlargement.
  - Left ventricular wall motion abnormalities.
  - Mitral regurgitation.
  - Pulmonary hypertension.
- Patients with HFrEF and new-onset angina will usually get referred for baseline coronary angiography.

- During subsequent follow-up of patients with HFrEF and CAD, certain findings may prompt a referral for a stress echocardiogram or a dobutamine stress echo:
  - New wall motion abnormalities on a resting echo.
  - Change in chest symptoms suggesting progression of coronary artery disease.
  - Decreased exercise tolerance.
  - Dyspnea on exertion.
  - Multiple hospital admissions for heart failure.
  - New Q waves on ECG.
  - New ST-segment, or T-wave abnormalities on ECG.
  - New ventricular arrhythmias.
- A rare patient may present to the echo lab following surgical left ventricular *reconstruction* of HFrEF.

  It is sometimes called endoventricular circular patch plasty, or a Dor procedure. The surgery restores left ventricular shape by surgical resection of abnormal anterior left ventricular wall segments.

Hillis LD, Smith PK, Anderson JL, et al. 2011 ACCF/AHA **guideline** for coronary artery bypass graft surgery. J Am Coll Cardiol. 2011;58:e123–e210.

Oh JK, Velazquez EJ, Menicanti L, et al. Influence of baseline left ventricular function on the clinical outcome of surgical **ventricular reconstruction** in patients with ischaemic cardiomyopathy. Eur Heart J. 2013;34:39–47.

Samad Z, Shaw LK, Phelan M, et al. Management and outcomes in patients with moderate or severe **functional mitral regurgitation** and severe left ventricular dysfunction. Eur Heart J. 2015;36:2733–2741.

Velazquez EJ. Does **imaging-guided selection** of patients with ischemic heart failure for high risk revascularization improve identification of those with the highest clinical benefit? Myocardial imaging should not exclude patients with ischemic heart failure from coronary revascularization. Circ Cardiovasc Imaging. 2012;5:271–279.

Velazquez EJ, Lee KL, Jones RH, et al. Coronary artery **bypass surgery** in patients with ischemic cardiomyopathy. N Engl J Med. 2016;374:1511–1520.

CORONARY FLOW RESERVE

- This is a technically challenging ultrasound technique (Fig. 7-4).
- It can provide prognostic information in coronary artery disease patients early after acute MI and help to identify nonviable myocardium.
- Technique: Coronary flow is increased by intravenous vasodilator infusion and compared to baseline.
- Coronary flow reserve is defined as the ratio between the increased diastolic coronary artery flow velocity and the resting diastolic flow velocity.

Pizzuto F, Voci P, Mariano E, et al. Assessment of flow velocity reserve by transthoracic Doppler echocardiography and venous adenosine infusion before and after left anterior descending coronary artery **stenting**. J Am Coll Cardiol. 2001;38:155–162.

Rigo F, Cortigiani L, Pasanisi E, et al. The additional **prognostic value** of coronary flow reserve on left anterior descending artery in patients with negative stress echo by wall motion criteria. A Transthoracic Vasodilator Stress Echocardiography Study. Am Heart J. 2006;151:124–130.

Saraste A, Koskenvuo J, Saraste M, et al. Coronary artery flow velocity profile measured by transthoracic Doppler echocardiography **predicts myocardial viability** after acute myocardial infarction. Heart. 2007;93:456–457.

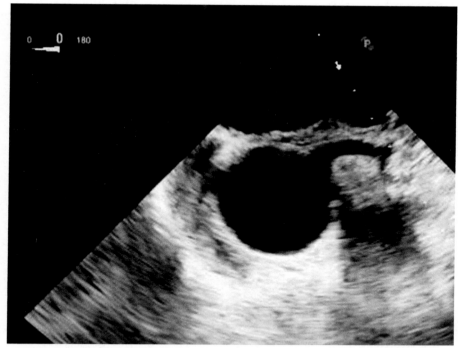

FIGURE 7-4. High resolution TEE image of the left main coronary artery. Doppler pitfall: Blood flow is perpendicular to the transducer, and it is not possible to measure coronary flow reserve. Color M-mode can still be used to time the flow.

ECHOCARDIOGRAPHY IN SCREENING FOR CORONARY ARTERY ABNORMALITIES

- Echocardiography is used in pediatrics to screen for coronary artery abnormalities.
- ALCAPA—anomalous left coronary artery from the pulmonary artery.
- The left main coronary artery can originate in the pulmonary artery.
- Doppler can show retrograde flow from the remaining normal-origin coronary arteries.

Hamada S, Yoshimura N, Takamiya M. Images in cardiovascular medicine. Noninvasive imaging of anomalous origin of the left coronary artery from the pulmonary artery. Circulation. 1998;97:219.

Lorber R, Srivastava S, Wilder TJ, et al. Anomalous aortic origin of coronary arteries in the young: echocardiographic evaluation with surgical correlation. JACC Cardiovasc Imaging. 2015;8:1239–1249.

Vaksmann G, Mauran P, Francart C, et al. Images in cardiovascular medicine. Noninvasive diagnosis of anomalous origin of the left main coronary artery from the pulmonary artery. Circulation. 1998;97:1869.

CORONARY CAMERAL FISTULAS

- A communication from a coronary artery to a ventricular cavity is manifested as *holodiastolic* color flow.

Padfield GJ. A case of coronary cameral fistula. Eur J Echocardiogr. 2009;10:718–720.

CORONARY ARTERY ORIGINS FROM THE WRONG SINUS

- Coronary artery origins are searched for in the parasternal short axis views at the level of the aortic leaflets.
- If a coronary artery is found on echo at the AV groove, it must be tracked back to its origin at the aortic root.
- Modified views are used to look for a left main artery originating from the right sinus of Valsalva.

Thankavel PP, Balakrishnan PL, Lemler MS, et al. Anomalous left main coronary artery origin from the right sinus of Valsalva (ALMCA): a novel echocardiographic screening method. Pediatr Cardiol. 2013;34:842–846.

The left main coronary was identified in the parasternal long-axis view between the aorta and pulmonary trunk. The angle of the left main coronary course was measured. In patients with ALMCA, the proximal course of the vessel was steeper as it coursed posteriorly. In contrast, the course was almost horizontal in patients with normal coronary origins. Based on these findings, a cutoff angle of 28 degrees is proposed. In the parasternal long-axis view, ALMCA can be identified by its anomalous proximal course. This screening method is reliable and increases the accuracy of transthoracic echocardiograms.

CORONARY ARTERY ANEURYSMS IN KAWASAKI DISEASE

- Kawasaki disease is a childhood disorder associated with coronary artery aneurysms.
- The aneurysms are found in the proximal portions of the coronary arteries.
- Screening for a suspected diagnosis in a child is done using transthoracic echo imaging.

*Brown LM, Duffy CE, Mitchell C, et al. A practical **guide** to pediatric coronary artery imaging with echocardiography. J Am Soc Echocardiogr. 2015;28:379–391.*

*Bruckheimer E, Bulbul Z, McCarthy P, et al. **Kawasaki** disease: coronary aneurysms in mother and son. Circulation. 1998;97:410–411.*

EXERCISE STRESS ECHOCARDIOGRAPHY

GUIDELINES

Pellikka PA, Arruda-Olson A, Chaudhry FA, et al. Guidelines for performance, interpretation, and application of stress echocardiography in ischemic heart disease: from the American Society of Echocardiography. J Am Soc Echocardiogr. 2020;33:1–41.

- *Comprehensive document.*
- *Download it at asecho.org.*
- *Learn what tables are available in this document and use them for future reference.*
- *Look at the illustration of curved M-mode strain imaging in LAD ischemia.*

- Exercise stress echo is performed on a treadmill or supine bicycle.
- A large amount of prognostic data is available.

- Guidelines (see above) and appropriate use criteria have been published.
- Gender differences and diabetes have been studied.
- Exercise echo is cost effective and has been favorably compared to nuclear techniques.
- Nuclear imaging is generally more sensitive, whereas echo imaging is more specific.
- A negative stress echo indicates low likelihood of adverse coronary outcomes.
- Both modalities are dependent on operator expertise.
- Advantages of echo include avoidance of radiation exposure and no need to return for subsequent nuclear imaging.
- Most of the following references are freely available as full-text articles that address the clinical utility of stress echocardiography.

Arruda-Olson AM, Juracan EM, Mahoney DW, et al. **Prognostic value** of exercise echocardiography in 5,798 patients: is there a gender difference? J Am Coll Cardiol. 2002;39:625–631.

Badruddin SM, Ahmad A, Mickelson J, et al. **Supine bicycle** versus post-treadmill exercise echocardiography in the detection of myocardial ischemia: a randomized single-blind crossover trial. J Am Coll Cardiol. 1999;33:1485–1490.

Beattie WS, Abdelnaem E, Wijeysundera DN, et al. A meta-analytic comparison of preoperative stress echocardiography and **nuclear scintigraphy imaging**. Anesth Analg. 2006;102:8–16.

Bouzas-Mosquera A, Peteiro J, Alvarez-Garcia N, et al. **Prediction of mortality** and major cardiac events by exercise echocardiography in patients with normal exercise electrocardiographic testing. J Am Coll Cardiol. 2009;53:1981–1990.

Cortigiani L, Borelli L, Raciti M, et al. Prediction of mortality by stress echocardiography in 2835 **diabetic** and 11305 nondiabetic patients. Circ Cardiovasc Imaging. 2015;8:e002757.

Gaur A, Yeon SB, Lewis CW, et al. **Valvular flow abnormalities** are often identified by a resting focused Doppler examination performed at the time of stress echocardiography. Am J Med. 2003;114:20–24.

Hoffmann U, Ferencik M, Udelson JE, et al. Prognostic value of noninvasive cardiovascular testing in patients with **stable chest pain**: insights from the promise trial (prospective multicenter imaging study for evaluation of chest pain). Circulation. 2017;135:2320–2332.

McCully RB, Roger VL, Mahoney DW, et al. Outcome after abnormal exercise echocardiography for patients with good exercise capacity: prognostic importance of the extent and severity of **exercise-related left ventricular dysfunction**. J Am Coll Cardiol. 2002;39:1345–1352.

McCully RB, Roger VL, Mahoney DW, et al. **Outcome after normal exercise** echocardiography and predictors of subsequent cardiac events: follow-up of 1,325 patients. J Am Coll Cardiol. 1998;31:144–149.

Mertes H, Erbel R, Nixdorff U, et al. Exercise echocardiography for the evaluation of patients **after nonsurgical coronary artery revascularization**. J Am Coll Cardiol. 1993;21:1087–1093.

Metz LD, Beattie M, Hom R, et al. The prognostic value of **normal exercise myocardial perfusion** imaging and exercise echocardiography: a meta-analysis. J Am Coll Cardiol. 2007;49:227–237.

Mieres JH, Gulati M, Bairey Merz N, et al. Role of noninvasive testing in the clinical evaluation of **women** with suspected ischemic heart disease: a consensus statement from the American Heart Association. Circulation. 2014;130:350–379.

Quinones MA, Verani MS, Haichin RM, et al. Exercise echocardiography **versus 201TI single-photon emission computed tomography** in evaluation of coronary artery disease. Analysis of 292 patients. Circulation. 1992;85:1026–1031.

Roger VL, Pellikka PA, Bell MR, et al. Sex and test verification bias. Impact on the **diagnostic value** of exercise echocardiography. Circulation. 1997;95:405–410.

Shaw LJ, Vasey C, Sawada S, et al. Impact of gender on risk stratification by exercise and dobutamine stress echocardiography: **long-term mortality** in 4234 women and 6898 men. Eur Heart J. 2005;26:447–456.

Sicari R, Pasanisi E, Venneri L, et al. Stress echo results **predict mortality**: a large-scale multicenter prospective international study. J Am Coll Cardiol. 2003;41:589–595.

Tischler MD, Niggel J. Exercise echocardiography in combined mild **mitral valve stenosis and regurgitation**. Echocardiography. 1993;10:453–457.

Tischler MD, Plehn JF. Applications of stress echocardiography: **beyond coronary** disease. J Am Soc Echocardiogr. 1995; 8:185–197.

Yao SS, Shah A, Bangalore S, et al. Transient ischemic **left ventricular cavity dilation** is a significant predictor of severe and extensive coronary artery disease and adverse outcome in patients undergoing stress echocardiography. J Am Soc Echocardiogr. 2007;20:352–358.

Zacharias K, Ahmed A, Shah BN, et al. Relative clinical and economic impact of **exercise echocardiography vs. exercise electrocardiography**, as first line investigation in patients without known coronary artery disease and new stable angina: a randomized prospective study. Eur Heart J Cardiovasc Imaging. 2017;18:195–202.

STRESS ECHO FOR EVALUATION OF DYSPNEA

- Exercise induced diastolic dysfunction can be found in patients with unexplained dyspnea.
- Exercise induced pulmonary hypertension can be found in subjects with a normal left ventricular ejection fraction.

Singhal S, Yousuf MA, Weintraub NL, et al. Use of bicycle exercise echocardiography for unexplained exertional dyspnea. Clin Cardiol. 2009;32:302–306.

Kane GC, Oh JK. Diastolic stress test for the evaluation of exertional dyspnea. Curr Cardiol Rep. 2012;14:359–365.

Ha JW, Choi D, Park S, et al. Determinants of exercise-induced pulmonary hypertension in patients with normal left ventricular ejection fraction. Heart. 2009;95:490–494.

SCANNING TIPS FOR DIASTOLIC STRESS ECHO

- E/e' ratio remains <10 in normal subjects during exercise.
- Exercise E velocity is measured as the heart is slowing down and E and A waves are no longer fused.
- Peak tricuspid regurgitation velocity does not exceed 3.1 m/s in normal subjects during exercise.
- Caution: Exercise e' may be affected by mitral annular calcium, left bundle branch block, or electronic pacemakers.
- Diastolic stunning may persist for hours after an abnormal stress test.
- Stress echo may unmask heart failure with preserved ejection fraction.

ECHOCARDIOGRAPHIC FINDINGS IN HEART FAILURE WITH PRESERVED EJECTION FRACTION

- Ejection fraction is normal, but stroke volume may be reduced.
- Stroke volume may not increase with exercise.
- Diastolic dysfunction is present.
- Left ventricular filling pressures are increased (E/e' >15).
- Pulmonary hypertension (TR >2.8 m/s).
- Abnormal myocardial strain.

- Increased left atrial size.
- Increased left ventricular wall thickness.

Ishii K, Imai M, Suyama T, et al. Exercise-induced post-ischemic left ventricular delayed relaxation or diastolic stunning: is it a reliable marker in detecting coronary artery disease? J Am Coll Cardiol. 2009;53:698–705.

Kane GC, Sachdev A, Villarraga HR, et al. Impact of age on pulmonary artery systolic pressures at rest and with exercise. Echo Res Pract. 2016;3:53–61.

Obokata M, Kane GC, Reddy YN, et al. Role of diastolic stress testing in the evaluation for heart failure with preserved ejection fraction: a simultaneous invasive-echocardiographic study. Circulation. 2017;135:825–838.

OFF-LABEL MYOCARDIAL PERFUSION

- The use of contrast for myocardial perfusion is currently off label.
- However, many echo labs around the world do look at myocardial perfusion along with wall motion analysis in the course of a stress echo.
- Following acute myocardial infarction, myocardial perfusion echocardiography may prove useful in the evaluation of myocardial viability.

Abdelmoneim SS, Dhoble A, Bernier M, et al. Quantitative myocardial contrast echocardiography during pharmacological stress for diagnosis of coronary artery disease: a systematic review and meta-analysis of diagnostic accuracy studies. Eur J Echocardiogr. 2009;10:813–825.

Ito H, Tomooka T, Sakai N, et al. Lack of myocardial perfusion immediately after successful thrombolysis. A predictor of poor recovery of left ventricular function in anterior myocardial infarction. Circulation. 1992;85:1699–1705.

VIDEOS

VIDEO 7-1. Ventricular septal rupture complicating acute myocardial infarction. The patient did not survive despite surgical repair.

VIDEO 7-2 (A–E). Ventricular septal rupture following acute myocardial infarction.

VIDEO 7-3 (A,B). Attempted patch closure of ventricular septal rupture following acute myocardial infarction.

VIDEO 7-4. Very large apical left ventricular aneurysm. There is spontaneous contrast in the left ventricular cavity, indicating stasis.

VIDEO 7-5 (A–E). Apical left ventricular aneurysm.

VIDEO 7-6. Apical left ventricular aneurysm. Preserved contractility of the basal portion of the left ventricle. Possible takotsubo—apical ballooning syndrome.

VIDEO 7-7. Apical left ventricular aneurysm. Multiple false tendons. No evident left ventricular thrombus.

VIDEO 7-8 (A,B). Apical aneurysm. Superimposed artifact. No thrombus.

VIDEO 7-9. Artifact. Normal apical wall motion. No thrombus.

VIDEO 7-10. Apical left ventricular aneurysm. Negative contrast changes shape; therefore, not a thrombus.

VIDEO 7-11. Apical left ventricular aneurysm. Contrast swirling. No thrombus.

VIDEO 7-12. Apical left ventricular aneurysm. Midventricular systolic cavity obstruction.

VIDEO 7-13 (A,B). Apical left ventricular pseudoaneurysm. Rupture "walled off" by intrapericardial thrombus.

VIDEO 7-14. Apical left ventricular thrombus. Normal papillary muscles at the base of the left ventricle.

VIDEO 7-15 (A–K). Apical left ventricular thrombus.

VIDEO 7-16. Calcified apical left ventricular thrombus.

VIDEO 7-17 (A,B). Apical right ventricular thrombus. Right ventricular infarction.

VIDEO 7-18. Apical left ventricular akinesis. "Door knob turning" sign.

VIDEO 7-19. Apical left ventricular akinesis.

VIDEO 7-20. Apical left ventricular dyskinesis.

VIDEO 7-21. Anterior infarction with basal septal hypertrophy, and systolic anterior motion of the mitral valve.

VIDEO 7-22. Peri infarct hypertrophy: Reactive basal septal hypertrophy triggered by adjacent mid and apical septal myocardial infarction.

VIDEO 7-23. Thinning of the apical walls.

VIDEO 7-24. Thinning, akinesis, and increased echogenicity of the interventricular septum due to an old anterior myocardial infarction. There is systolic left ventricular dysfunction and biatrial enlargement. There is apical tethering of the mitral valve, with localized calcification at the papillary muscle tip. Note that there is no secundum atrial septal defect. The thin membrane of the intact fossa ovalis simply does not reflect any ultrasound back at the transducer.

VIDEO 7-25. Aneurysm and scarring (increased echogenicity) of the basal inferoseptal wall. There is a restraining chorda/false tendon from the aneurysm wall to the papillary muscles.

VIDEO 7-26. Absence of myocardial thickening at the midportion of the interventricular septum.

VIDEO 7-27. Global left ventricular hypokinesis.

VIDEO 7-28. Dilated left ventricle. Lack of thickening of the mid and apical inferior wall. Akinesis and typical "scooped out" appearance of the basal inferior wall. Hypokinesis of the anterior wall. Subtle systolic expansion of the left atrial appendage.

VIDEO 7-29. Akinetic basal and mid-anterolateral walls. Circumflex coronary artery occlusion.

VIDEO 7-30. Apical lateral wall akinesis.

VIDEO 7-31. Akinetic basal and mid-inferolateral wall.

VIDEO 7-32. Basal inferolateral wall akinesis. Apical tethering of the mitral valve.

VIDEO 7-33. Prominent apical lateral left ventricular wall trabeculations that should not be mistaken for a thrombus.

VIDEO 7-34 (A,B). Apical artifact that resembles a thrombus. Normal endocardial motion partly hidden by the artifact.

VIDEO 7-35 (A–D). A false tendon should not be mistaken for the edge of an apical thrombus. A false tendon typically begins at a characteristic triangular-shaped trabeculation.

VIDEO 7-36 (A–C). False tendon—typical triangular anchoring.

VIDEO 7-37 (A,B). Apical left ventricular akinesis. Prominent apical trabeculations. Apical thrombus demonstrated with contrast.

VIDEO 7-38. A previously stretched taut false tendon became highly mobile after a TAVR.

VIDEO 7-39. Large basal inferior left ventricular wall aneurysm. The large size of this aneurysmal dilatation of the basal inferior wall is unusual after inferior myocardial infarction. It can be associated with ventricular septal rupture. In some cases there may be a question as to whether it is a true aneurysm or a pseudoaneurysm.

VIDEO 7-40 (A,B). Basal inferior aneurysm. Apical tethering of the mitral valve. Taut mitral chordae across the mouth of the aneurysm. Small fibrinous pericardial effusion.

VIDEO 7-41. Walled-off inferior wall rupture is difficult to distinguish from a large inferior aneurysm.

VIDEO 7-42. Akinesis of the basal and mid-inferior left ventricular wall. Calcifications of mitral chordae and papillary muscles suggest that this is an old inferior infarction. The incidentally noted false tendon close to the apex may rarely cause a murmur. In this patient, mitral regurgitation is a more likely cause of an apical systolic murmur.

VIDEO 7-43. Midventricular inferior and inferolateral wall akinesis.

VIDEO 7-44 (A,B). Basal inferior and inferolateral wall akinesis.

VIDEO 7-45. Basal and mid-inferior left ventricular wall akinesis.

VIDEO 7-46. Inferior myocardial infarction. Lack of systolic thickening of the basal and mid-inferior wall. Normal thickening of the anterior wall.

VIDEO 7-47. Basal and mid-inferior left ventricular wall akinesis.

VIDEO 7-48. Basal and mid-inferior thinning and akinesis.

VIDEO 7-49. Basal inferior left ventricular wall dyskinesis.

VIDEO 7-50. Basal inferior left ventricular wall akinesis and scar (increased reflectivity).

VIDEO 7-51. Apical and mid-inferior left ventricular wall akinesis.

VIDEO 7-52. Akinetic inferior left ventricular wall. The akinesis extends to the inferior right ventricular wall.

VIDEO 7-53. Akinesis, thinning, and increased reflectivity (indicating scar) of the basal and mid-interventricular septum.

VIDEO 7-54. Akinetic mid-inferior and mid-inferoseptal wall.

VIDEO 7-55. Basal inferoseptal left ventricular wall akinesis.

VIDEO 7-56. Basal inferoseptal left ventricular aneurysm. Mitral prosthetic ring dehiscence.

VIDEO 7-57. Inferior right ventricular wall akinesis.

VIDEO 7-58. Basal and mid-inferolateral left ventricular wall akinesis.

VIDEO 7-59. Basal and mid-anterolateral left ventricular wall akinesis.

VIDEO 7-60 (A–C). Inferior akinesis.

VIDEO 7-61 (A–C). Inferior left ventricular infarction with extension to the inferior right ventricular wall.

VIDEO 7-62. Right ventricular infarction.

VIDEO 7-63. Apical anterior left ventricular wall akinesis.

VIDEO 7-64 (A,B). Anterior and apical inferior wall akinesis (LAD distribution).

VIDEO 7-65. Basal and mid-anteroseptal wall akinesis in total LAD occlusion.

VIDEO 7-66. Mid-anteroseptal wall akinesis.

VIDEO 7-67. Apical right ventricular pacing. Apical septal dyskinesis.

VIDEO 7-68. Anterior wall akinesis.

VIDEO 7-69. Basal and mid-anteroseptal left ventricular wall akinesis.

VIDEO 7-70. Basal anteroseptal thinning and akinesis.

VIDEO 7-71 (A,B). Basal inferoseptal thinning and akinesis.

VIDEO 7-72. Apical lateral wall akinesis.

VIDEO 7-73. Anterolateral wall akinesis.

VIDEO 7-74. Basal and mid-anterolateral wall akinesis. Effect of a PVC.

VIDEO 7-75. Normal baseline wall motion. Effect of a PVC.

VIDEO 7-76. Localized thinning and dyskinesis of the apical right ventricular free wall.

VIDEO 7-77. Normal takeoff of the left main coronary artery at 3 o'clock.

VIDEO 7-78. Left main coronary artery.

VIDEO 7-79 (A,B). Anomalous left coronary artery from the pulmonary artery.

VIDEO 7-80 (A,B). Normal right coronary artery.

VIDEO 7-81 (A,B). Right coronary ostium at 11 o'clock.

VIDEO 7-82. Right coronary artery at 6 o'clock.

VIDEO 7-83. Right and left coronary origins.

VIDEO 7-84. Coronary artery seen intermittently as two parallel lines.

VIDEO 7-85 (A,B). Coronary artery seen intermittently over the aortic leaflets.

VIDEO 7-86. Large, partly thrombosed aneurysm of the left main coronary artery.

VIDEO 7-87 (A,B). Beam width artifact. A coronary artery appears out of place.

VIDEO 7-88. Coronary artery seen intermittently over the interventricular septum.

VIDEO 7-89 (A–D). Coronary artery flow.

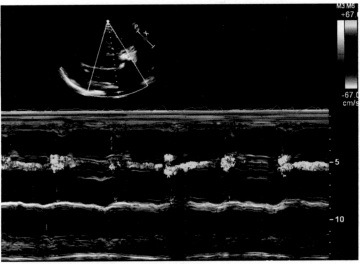

FIGURE 7-5. Timing of coronary artery flow.

VIDEO 7-90. Color flow of mild pulmonic valve regurgitation originating very close to the area where the proximal left main coronary artery can be visualized. Timing the color flow with color M-mode can be useful. Pulmonic regurgitation is limited to diastole. Coronary flow occurs both in systole and in diastole. Unusually prominent coronary artery color flow can be a clue to possible left main coronary artery stenosis. In this case the flow represents pulmonic regurgitation.

VIDEO 7-91. Coronary artery flow that was initially misinterpreted as paravalvular aortic prosthesis regurgitation.

VIDEO 7-92. Flash technique for myocardial perfusion.

VIDEO 7-93. Wall motion in left bundle branch block.

VIDEO 7-94. Attenuation of the basal lateral wall.

VIDEO 7-95. Cardiogenic shock due to extensive right ventricular infarction.

VIDEO 7-96. Epicardial coronary artery flow.

AREA CALCULATION IN ATRIAL FIBRILLATION

- If the heart rhythm is irregular, the LVOT velocities and the valve stenosis velocities will be affected by the length of the cardiac cycle.
- It is customary, and recommended, to *average* 5 to 10 fluctuating velocities when calculating the severity of aortic stenosis in atrial fibrillation.
- It is also possible to *match the RR* intervals of the LVOT and stenosis signals being used for the calculation.
- The aortic valve area calculated by the *highest velocity ratio* was found to be acceptable in the reference below.
- The guidelines should be checked for the latest recommendations.

Alsidawi S, Khan S, Pislaru SV, et al. Aortic valve hemodynamics in atrial fibrillation: should the highest Doppler signal be used to estimate severity of aortic stenosis? Echocardiography. 2018;35:869–871.

AORTIC VALVE RESISTANCE

"28 × square root of the mean gradient ÷ area."
- A measure of aortic stenosis: less affected by changes in flow.

Bermejo J, García-Fernández MA, Torrecilla EG, et al. Effects of dobutamine on Doppler echocardiographic indexes of aortic stenosis. J Am Coll Cardiol. 1996;28:1206–1213.

A low dose dobutamine protocol was performed in patients with aortic stenosis.
- *At peak flow:*
  - *Valve area increased by 28%.*
  - *Valve resistance decreased by 4%.*

VALVULOARTERIAL IMPEDANCE

"Systolic blood pressure + mean gradient ÷ stroke volume index."
- Excessive load on the left ventricle from combined:
  - Aortic stenosis.
  - Resistance from the aorta.
- A value >3.5 identifies patients with a poor outcome.

Hachicha Z, Dumesnil JG, Pibarot P. Usefulness of the valvuloarterial impedance to predict adverse outcome in asymptomatic aortic stenosis. J Am Coll Cardiol. 2009;54:1003–1011.

RIGHT SUBCLAVIAN ARTERY STENOSIS

- A high-velocity signal originating from a stenotic right subclavian artery can be mistaken for an aortic stenosis jet.
- Differences in the shapes of the jets obtained from an apical and right supraclavicular position should indicate different origins of these two high-velocity systolic signals.
- Correct identification of the origin of each signal is possible with pulsed-wave Doppler recordings of the subclavian artery, and with high pulse-repetition-frequency pulsed Doppler interrogation of the aortic valve.

- TEE may be required to further image the stenotic aortic valve with planimetry if subclavian artery stenosis is suspected.

Otto CM, Miyake-Hull CY, Gardner CJ, et al. Subclavian artery stenosis masquerading as prosthetic aortic stenosis: a potential source of confusion in Doppler evaluation of aortic valve disease. J Am Soc Echocardiogr. 1992;5:459–462.

SUBAORTIC STENOSIS

- Rare patients can have a "washer-like" membrane in the left ventricular outflow.
- This causes a fixed (not dynamic) obstruction below the aortic valve.
- Caution: It may be missed by an inexperienced sonographer.
- Over the years, there may be progressive damage to the aortic valve from the turbulent flow. As a result, these patients have variable degrees of aortic valve regurgitation.
- Surgical resection of the obstructive membrane is usually advised.

Aboulhosn J, Child JS. Echocardiographic evaluation of congenital left ventricular outflow obstruction. Echocardiography. 2015;32 Suppl 2:S140–S147.

SUPRAVALVULAR AORTIC STENOSIS

- This is a rare cause of downstream obstruction to left ventricular outflow.
- The aortic leaflet opening is usually normal. As a result, the aortic component of the second heart sound is audible (not decreased).
- There may be discreet membrane-like obstruction to forward flow in the proximal ascending aorta.
- Other patients with this hemodynamic abnormality have a smaller-than-normal (hypoplastic) aorta.
- It is important to image the entire aorta with additional modalities such as CT aortography or MRI.

www.omim.org

The Online Mendelian Inheritance in Man Database. Search for "Williams Beuren syndrome" and for "maternal rubella".

SHONE COMPLEX

- This is a rare congenital cardiac malformation characterized by four serial obstructive lesions of the left side of the heart:
  - Supravalvular mitral membrane.
  - Parachute mitral valve.
  - Muscular or membranous subaortic stenosis.
  - Coarctation of the aorta.

Aslam S, Khairy P, Shohoudi A, et al. Shone complex: an under-recognized congenital heart disease with substantial morbidity in adulthood. Can J Cardiol. 2017;33:253–259.

VIDEOS

VIDEO 8-1 (A,B). Normal trileaflet aortic valve.

VIDEO 8-2 (A,B). Mild thickening of the aortic leaflet commissures.

VIDEO 8-3. Slitlike aortic leaflet opening.

VIDEO 8-4. Artifactual duplication of the aortic leaflets.

VIDEO 8-5. Post-PVC increase in aortic stenosis gradient.

VIDEO 8-6. Nodule of Arantius on the noncoronary aortic cusp.

VIDEO 8-7 (A–C). Nodule of Arantius on the left coronary aortic cusp.

VIDEO 8-8. Beam width/slice thickness artifact. Aortic valve sclerosis. Mobile aortic leaflets. Superimposed immobile calcifications.

VIDEO 8-9 (A–C). Subaortic membrane.

VIDEO 8-10. TEE anatomy: The noncoronary aortic cusp is "bisected" by the interatrial septum.

NOTES

CHAPTER 9

Bicuspid Aortic Valve

ECHO FEATURES OF BICUSPID AORTIC VALVES

- Definition
  - Bicuspid aortic valve: two instead of three semilunar aortic valve cusps.
  - There are also rare patients with unicuspid and quadricuspid aortic valves.
- Cusp nomenclature
  - The *conjoined* cusp is usually wider than normal and contains a raphe.
  - Raphe: a ridge that extends from the aortic wall to the commissure of the conjoined cusp.
- Raphe height variants
  - No evident raphe, just a "fishmouth" systolic opening.
  - Shallow, difficult-to-image raphe.
  - Classic thick visible raphe.
  - Unusually tall raphe—rising as high as the free edge of the leaflets.
- Over time, the raphe may become calcified. Calcification is manifested on echo by acoustic shadowing past the raphe.
- Classification:
  - Type 1: Fusion of the right and left coronary cusp (larger sinus diameter) (70%–86% incidence).
  - Type 2: Fusion of the right and noncoronary cusp (associated tubular ascending aorta and dilated arch) (12%–28% incidence).
  - Type 3: Fusion of the left and noncoronary cusp (rare incidence).
- Imaging:
  - Parasternal long axis (PLAX) view provides the first clue to the presence of a bicuspid valve.
  - Asymmetric diastolic leaflet closure line located on an "outside third" of the sinus of Valsalva (Fig. 9-1).
  - Systolic doming.
  - Diastolic prolapse.

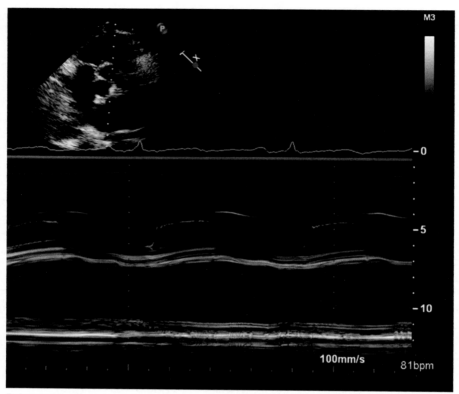

FIGURE 9-1. Bicuspid aortic valve. Eccentric leaflet closure.

- Short axis (SAX) view is used for definitive diagnosis. Sometimes transesophageal echocardiography (TEE) is needed for confirmation.
- Diastole may fool you: The closed valve may look perfectly normal on echo when a nonthickened raphe is present.
- Look for a thicker than normal, partly unseparated raphe in systole.
- Look for the systolic "fishmouth" opening.
- A commissure line may continue "past the center" without bending.
- A commissure may violate the 10–2–6 o'clock location.
- When the intercoronary (right to left) commissure is abnormal (type 1), the systolic opening has a *horizontal* orientation.
- When the right-to-noncoronary commissure is abnormal (type 2), the systolic opening has a *vertical* orientation.
- Doppler evaluation of the systolic gradient in bicuspid aortic valves:
  - The maximum instantaneous Doppler gradient is typically higher than a peak-to-peak gradient measured by catheterization.
  - The *mean* Doppler gradient is closer to the peak-to-peak gradient measured by catheterization.
  - The discrepancy is explained in some cases by the presence of pressure recovery.

- Direct planimetry of 2D and 3D echo images should be done when feasible (making sure the smallest possible, "mouth of the volcano," true stenosis orifice is used).
- In children with a stenotic bicuspid, or a unicuspid aortic valve, the presence of left ventricular hypertrophy indicates significant valve obstruction.
- Bicuspid aortic valve is associated with coarctation of the aorta.

Espinola-Zavaleta N, Muñoz-Castellanos L, Attié F, et al. Anatomic three-dimensional echocardiographic correlation of bicuspid aortic valve. J Am Soc Echocardiogr. 2003;16:46–53.

Michelena HI, Khanna AD, Mahoney D, et al. Incidence of **aortic complications** in patients with bicuspid aortic valves. JAMA. 2011;306:1104–1112.

Muraru D, Badano LP, Vannan M, et al. Assessment of aortic valve complex by three-dimensional echocardiography: a framework for its effective application in clinical practice. Eur Heart J Cardiovasc Imaging. 2012;13:541–555.

Schaefer BM, Lewin MB, Stout KK, et al. The bicuspid aortic valve: an integrated phenotypic classification of **leaflet morphology** and aortic root shape. Heart. 2008;94:1634–1638.

Siu SC, Silversides K. Bicuspid aortic valve disease. J Am Coll Cardiol. 2010;55:2789–2800.
Review article.

Tadros TM, Klein MD, Shapira OM. Ascending aortic dilatation associated with bicuspid aortic valve. Pathophysiology, **molecular biology**, and clinical implications. Circulation. 2009;119:880–890.

Verma S, Siu SC. **Aortic dilatation** in patients with bicuspid aortic valve. N Engl J Med. 2014;370:1920–1929.

UNICUSPID AORTIC VALVE

- Clinical features in adults:
  - Aortic stenosis was the predominant associated hemodynamic lesion.
  - On average, this required surgical intervention during the third decade of life.
  - The valves are unicommissural with a posteriorly positioned commissural attachment.
  - Coexisting dilatation of the aortic annulus was found in almost half of patients.

Novaro GM, Mishra M, Griffin BP. Incidence and echocardiographic features of congenital unicuspid aortic valve in an adult population. J Heart Valve Dis. 2003;12:674–678.

Noly PE, Basmadjian L, Bouhout I, et al. New insights into unicuspid aortic valve disease in adults: not just a subtype of bicuspid aortic valves. Can J Cardiol. 2016;32:110–116.

COARCTATION OF THE AORTA

- The embryologic aorta begins as six paired arches.
  - The right fourth arch becomes the right subclavian artery.
  - The left fourth arch becomes the aortic arch.
- Improper development results in localized shelf-like narrowing of the descending aorta just past the left subclavian artery, near the location of the ductus arteriosus.
- 2D echo in the adult laboratory is used to image the long axis of the aorta from the suprasternal views.

- Color Doppler looks for flow acceleration and turbulence at the narrowing, and for the rate of narrowing of the cone of acceleration.
- In patients with coarctation, it is necessary to use the expanded Bernoulli equation:
  - $(4V^2$ distal$) - (4V^2$ proximal$)$.
  - The proximal velocity is included in the gradient calculation.
- Severe coarctation has a "sawtooth" CW pattern created by a constant gradient in systole and in diastole.
- Subcostal Doppler interrogation of the aorta in severe coarctation:
  - Delayed, decreased, gradual systolic upstroke that continues into diastole with persistence of turbulent flow.
  - Every patient with hypertension, left ventricular hypertrophy, or a bicuspid aortic valve should be evaluated by echo for coarctation.
- Coarctation is associated with:
  - Bicuspid aortic valve.
  - Ventricular septal defect.
  - Patent ductus arteriosus.
  - Aortic arch hypoplasia.
- Prenatal diagnosis of coarctation remains difficult.
- Most patients present in infancy with:
  - Absent, delayed, or reduced femoral pulses.
  - A supine arm-leg blood pressure gradient (>20 mm Hg).
  - A murmur due to rapid blood flow across the coarctation.
  - Bicuspid aortic valve.
- Adequate and timely diagnosis is crucial for good prognosis.
- Early treatment is associated with lower risks of long-term morbidity and mortality:
  - Surgical resection is the treatment of choice in neonates, infants, and young children.
  - In older children (>25 kg) and adults, transcatheter treatment is the treatment of choice.
- Patients with coarctation have a reduced life expectancy.
  - They have an increased risk of cardiovascular sequelae later in life, despite adequate relief of the stenosis in the aorta.
- Follow-up:
  - Left ventricular thickness and function.
  - Aortic valve function.
  - Blood pressure.
  - Morphology of the aorta.

Dijkema EJ, Leiner T, Grotenhuis HB. Diagnosis, imaging and clinical management of aortic coarctation. Heart. 2017;103: 1148–1155.

- The second heart sound may be *decreased* in patients with aortic regurgitation that is being caused by restricted leaflet motion in combined aortic stenosis and aortic regurgitation (AS/AR).
- AS/AR murmurs have a to-and-fro bellows quality with a decreased A2 between the harsh systolic ejection murmur and the blowing decrescendo diastolic regurgitation murmur.
- **Chronic** severe aortic regurgitation has numerous *eponyms* for physical findings caused by the wide pulse pressure:
  - Corrigan pulse: prominent pulsations of the carotid arteries.
  - Bisferiens pulse: double systolic arterial impulse—the so-called twice-beating heart.
  - De Musset sign: head nodding with each heartbeat.
  - Duroziez sign: systolic and diastolic femoral artery bruit.
  - Hill sign: accentuated leg systolic pressure with >40 mm Hg difference from the brachial artery systolic pressure.
  - Muller sign: pulsation of the uvula with each heartbeat.
  - Palmar click: palpable systolic flushing of the palms.
  - Quincke pulse: cyclic reddening and blanching of the nail capillaries.
  - Traube sign: loud "pistol shot" sound heard over the femoral artery.
  - Water hammer pulse: brisk femoral pulsation similar to that felt with a water hammer—a Victorian toy. The water hammer was a glass tube filled partly with water or mercury in a vacuum. The water or mercury produced a slapping impact when the glass tube was turned over.
- Clinical findings in **acute** severe aortic regurgitation:
  - The left ventricle is *not* dilated.
  - The left ventricle appears hyperdynamic on echo.
  - Forward stroke volume is *decreased*.
  - There is no systolic hypertension.
  - Pulse pressure is not widened.
  - The first heart sound is decreased.
- Echocardiographic correlate of a decreased first heart sound in acute severe aortic regurgitation: mitral valve preclosure and diastolic mitral regurgitation (Figs. 10-2 and 10-3).

Stout KK, Verrier ED. **Acute** *valvular regurgitation. Circulation. 2009;119:3232–3241.*

- *Acute severe valvular regurgitation is a surgical emergency.*
- *Accurate and timely diagnosis can be difficult.*
- *Cardiovascular collapse is a common presentation.*
- *Examination findings to suggest acute regurgitation may be subtle.*
- *The clinical presentation may be nonspecific.*
- *The presentation of acute valvular regurgitation may be mistaken for other acute conditions, such as sepsis, pneumonia, or nonvalvular heart failure.*

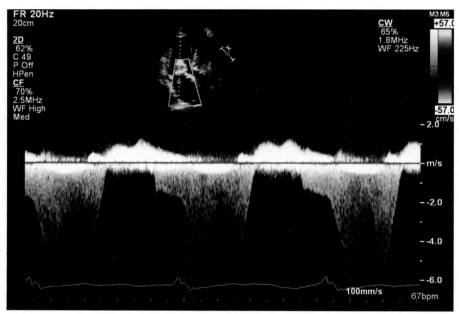

FIGURE 10-2. Diastolic mitral regurgitation in acute severe aortic regurgitation.

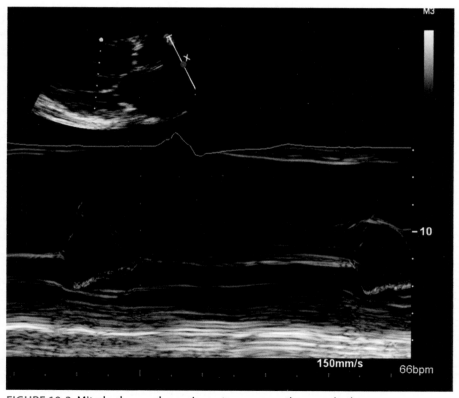

FIGURE 10-3. Mitral valve preclosure in acute severe aortic regurgitation.

- Three components of the aortic regurgitation jet on color flow in PLAX:
  - Flow convergence.
  - Vena contracta.
  - Jet height/width.
- Calculations:
  - Regurgitant flow rate: $2\pi r^2 \times$ aliasing velocity.
  - EROA: Regurgitant flow rate ÷ peak AR velocity.
  - Regurgitant volume: EROA × AR VTI.
- Findings in *severe chronic* AR:
  - EROA >0.30 cm^2.
  - Regurgitant volume >60 cc.
  - Jet height/LVOT ratio >65%.
  - Severely dilated spherical left ventricle.
  - Diastolic flow reversal in the descending aorta (Fig. 10-4).
  - Dense AR Doppler signal.
  - Short AR Doppler pressure half-time <200 ms.
- 2D morphology to define the *mechanism* of AR:
  - Sinotubular enlargement and dilatation of the ascending aorta.
  - Dilatation of the sinuses of Valsalva and sinotubular junction.

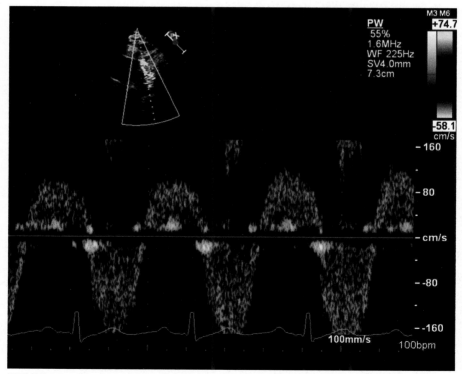

FIGURE 10-4. Severe aortic regurgitation. Diastolic flow reversal in the descending aorta.

- Dilatation of the ventriculo-arterial junction (LVOT annulus).
- Perforation.
- Prolapse.
- Leaflet restriction (thickening/calcification).
- M-mode findings:
  - Diastolic fluttering of the anterior mitral leaflet.
  - Early diastolic dip of the interventricular septum.
  - Mitral valve preclosure.
- Indications for echo evaluation:
  - Confirmation of diagnosis when the physical exam is equivocal.
  - Determination of severity or cause of AR.
  - New or changing symptoms in known AR.
  - Determining left ventricular size and function in severe AR.
  - Measurement of aortic root size.

Caution: In patients with combined mitral stenosis and significant aortic regurgitation, mitral pressure half time may be shortened by the AR—resulting in overestimation of mitral stenosis area.

- Left ventricular end-diastolic pressure (LVEDP) can be calculated using the Bernoulli equation in patients with AR:
  - The end-diastolic velocity is used to calculate a gradient ($4V^2$).
  - LVEDP = diastolic BP minus this gradient.
- Look for consistency: Mitral inflow will show a restrictive pattern with elevated LVEDP.

Nishimura RA, Vonk GD, Rumberger JA, et al. **Semiquantitation** of aortic regurgitation by different Doppler echocardiographic techniques and comparison with ultrafast computed tomography. Am Heart J. 1992;124:995–1001.

Oh JK, Hatle LK, Sinak LJ, et al. Characteristic Doppler echocardiographic pattern of **mitral inflow** velocity in severe aortic regurgitation. J Am Coll Cardiol. 1989;14:1712–1717.

Perry GJ, Helmcke F, Nanda NC, et al. Evaluation of aortic insufficiency by Doppler **color flow** mapping. J Am Coll Cardiol. 1987;9:952–959.

Samstad SO, Hegrenaes L, Skjaerpe T, et al. **Half time** of the diastolic aortoventricular pressure difference by continuous wave Doppler ultrasound: a measure of the severity of aortic regurgitation? Br Heart J. 1989;61:336–343.

Tribouilloy CM, Enriquez-Sarano M, Fett SL, et al. Application of the proximal flow convergence method to calculate the effective **regurgitant orifice** area in aortic regurgitation. J Am Coll Cardiol. 1998;32:1032–1039.

VIDEOS

VIDEO 10-1. Aortic regurgitation jet with proximal flow convergence.

VIDEO 10-2 (A,B). Wide aortic regurgitation jet.

VIDEO 10-3. Trace aortic regurgitation.

VIDEO 10-4. Severe aortic regurgitation due to aortic leaflet thickening and retraction.

VIDEO 10-5 (A,B). Central aortic regurgitant orifice.

VIDEO 10-6. Rheumatic aortic valve disease.

VIDEO 10-7. Aortic regurgitation and a mitral bioprosthesis. Useful Pedoff scanning tip: The aortic diastolic velocity on CW will always exceed the mitral CW velocity. Higher diastolic "driving" pressure from the aorta than from the LA.

VIDEO 10-8. The amount of aortic regurgitation increases with longer cardiac cycles. Systole duration is unchanged. Duration of diastole is visibly affected.

VIDEO 10-9. Aortic regurgitation jet impinging on the anterior mitral leaflet. Note: There is a misconception that diastolic fluttering of the anterior mitral leaflet on M-mode correlates with severity of regurgitation. It does not. Conversely, the auscultatory equivalent—the Austin Flint murmur does correlate with regurgitation severity. This low frequency mid to late diastolic murmur is found in patients with severe chronic aortic regurgitation.

VIDEO 10-10. Instead of impinging on the anterior mitral leaflet, the aortic regurgitation jet seems to pull it by a Venturi effect.

VIDEO 10-11 (A,B). Subaortic membrane.

NOTES

CHAPTER 11

Mitral Regurgitation

PRIMARY MITRAL REGURGITATION

- Definition: Mitral valve apparatus is directly affected.
- Examples: Prolapse, flail leaflet, endocarditis.
- The Carpentier classification is useful for understanding etiology as well as therapeutic approaches.
  - **Type I:** Normal leaflet size and motion, with the mitral regurgitation due to leaflet perforation or congenital clefts.
  - **Type II:** Excessive leaflet motion with prolapse or flail leaflets.
  - **Type IIIa:** Leaflet restriction in diastole, most commonly seen in rheumatic disease.

El Sabbagh A, Reddy YNV, Nishimura RA. Mitral Valve Regurgitation in the contemporary era: insights into diagnosis, management, and future directions. JACC Cardiovasc Imaging. 2018;11:628–643.

SECONDARY OR FUNCTIONAL MITRAL REGURGITATION

- Definition: The actual cause of the mitral regurgitation resides in the ventricle (not in the valve).
  - Mitral leaflets and chordae are structurally normal.
  - There is an imbalance between closing and tethering forces on the valve.
  - It is caused by alterations in LV geometry.
- Examples: mitral annular dilatation due to dilated cardiomyopathy, dilated left atrium, chronic atrial fibrillation.
- As the mitral annulus dilates, the coaptive surface decreases (less and less of the leaflet tips are touching).
- Apical tethering can be measured as tenting area (performed in mid-systole when the area is at its smallest).
- Leaflet tethering is often asymmetric in ischemic cardiomyopathies.
- In these cases of unbalanced tethering due to regional wall motion abnormalities:
  - The mitral regurgitation color flow jet is directed *away* from the relatively prolapsing leaflet.

- It is directed *toward* the relatively restricted leaflet.
- Initially left ventricular function becomes hyperdynamic.
- Global longitudinal strain may detect subtle left ventricular dysfunction.

Asgar AW, Mack MJ, Stone GW. *Secondary mitral regurgitation* in heart failure: pathophysiology, prognosis, and therapeutic considerations. J Am Coll Cardiol. 2015;65:1231–1248.

COLOR FLOW IN MITRAL REGURGITATION

- Jet area depicts blood flow velocities. This is not blood volume. It is a spatial display of velocities.
- Simply increasing left ventricular systolic "driving" pressure will increase the jet area with the same regurgitant orifice.
- Entrainment: A central mitral regurgitation jet will "pull in" (entrain) innocent bystander red blood cells that are already in the left atrium, exaggerating the apparent degree of regurgitation on color flow. When subjectively estimating the degree of regurgitation, one may want to "mentally downgrade" the severity.
- Coanda: An impinging eccentric mitral regurgitation jet creates the opposite dilemma: It may underrepresent the true severity of the regurgitation.

VENA CONTRACTA TECHNIQUE

- The transducer should be tilted so that PISA, vena contracta, and jet area can be identified.
- Zoom mode is preferred.
- Color flow sector should be kept to a minimum to optimize resolution.

MITRAL VALVE PROLAPSE

- One or both leaflets buckle back into the left atrium, characteristically in mid- to late systole. The plane of the mitral annulus is used for reference. The displacement should be >2 mm in either the PLAX or apical long-axis view (Fig. 11-1).
- Look for abnormalities of mitral valve chordae (ruptured, elongated, asymmetrically tethered, thickened, infected).
- Coronary artery disease can be complicated by prolapse. There may be regional left ventricular motion abnormalities that unbalance leaflet closure.
- A "Barlow" valve is >5 mm thick (myxomatous).
- Mitral valve prolapse can be a manifestation of Marfan syndrome or other connective tissue disorders.
- Chest wall abnormalities such as pectus excavatum, or scoliosis of the spine, can press and deform the mitral annulus and create prolapse.
- On auscultation there is a mid-systolic click.
- Surgical repair of a prolapsing middle scallop of the posterior mitral leaflet consists of the following:
  - Wedge resection of the prolapsing scallop.

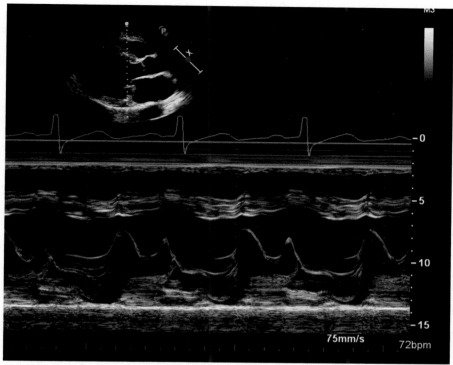

FIGURE 11-1. Classic M-mode of mitral valve prolapse.

- Sliding annuloplasty (joining the remaining tissue and annulus with sutures).
- Sewing a supporting prosthetic ring to the native annulus.
- Imaging:
  - Anterior leaflet prolapse can be mistakenly falsely overdiagnosed in the apical four-chamber view because of the mitral valve's convexo-concave saddle shape.
  - PISA measurement of mitral effective regurgitant orifice area (ERO) may overestimate the severity of mitral regurgitation. It is important to calculate the regurgitant volume (ERO × VTI).
  - Example: If ERO is 0.4 cm^2 then VTI has to be 150 cm for the regurgitant volume to reach 60 cc.

PICKELHAUBE SIGN

"Spiked configuration of the lateral annular tissue Doppler velocities in mitral valve prolapse."

- Tugging of the posteromedial papillary muscle in mid-systole by myxomatous prolapsing leaflets causes the adjacent posterobasal left ventricular wall to be pulled sharply toward the apex.

- This results in a spiked configuration of the lateral annular tissue Doppler velocities: Pickelhaube spiked helmet sign.
- This mechanical traction of the papillary muscles and posterolateral left ventricular wall is considered arrhythmogenic.

Avierinos JF, Gersh BJ, Melton LJ III, et al. Natural history of **asymptomatic** mitral valve prolapse in the community. Circulation. 2002;106:1355–1361.

Freed LA, Levy D, Levine RA, et al. Prevalence and clinical **outcome** of mitral-valve prolapse. N Engl J Med. 1999;341:1–7.

Kehl DW, Rader F, Siegel RJ. Echocardiographic features and clinical outcomes of **flail** mitral leaflet without severe mitral regurgitation. J Am Soc Echocardiogr. 2017;30:1162–1168.

Marks AR, Choong CY, Sanfilippo AJ, et al. Identification of **high-risk** and low-risk subgroups of patients with mitral-valve prolapse. N Engl J Med. 1989;320:1031–1036.

Muthukumar L, Rahman F, Jan MF, et al. The **Pickelhaube** sign: novel echocardiographic risk marker for malignant mitral valve prolapse syndrome. JACC Cardiovasc Imaging. 2017;10:1078–1080.

Nishimura RA, McGoon MD, Shub C, et al. Echocardiographically documented mitral-valve prolapse. Long-term **follow-up** of 237 patients. N Engl J Med. 1985;313:1305–1309.

MITRAL ANNULUS DISJUNCTION

- A floppy mitral valve may develop from hypermobility of the valve apparatus.
- Disjunction of the mitral annulus fibrosus is an anatomic variation in the morphology of the annulus.
- There is a separation between the atrial wall–mitral valve junction and the left ventricular attachment.
- This may be evident in the parasternal long axis images:
  - The posterior mitral leaflet buckles up into the left atrial cavity in systole.
  - At the same time there is hypermobility of the adjoining posterior mitral annulus in the opposite direction toward the left ventricular apex.

Hutchins GM, Moore GW, Skoog DK. The association of floppy mitral valve with disjunction of the mitral annulus fibrosus. N Engl J Med. 1986;314:535–540.

CHAPTER 12

Mitral Stenosis

GUIDELINES

Baumgartner H, Hung J, Bermejo J, et al. *Echocardiographic assessment of valve stenosis: EAE/ASE recommendations for clinical practice. Eur J Echocardiogr. 2009;10:1–25.*

■ Basic measurements of mitral stenosis severity are explained and illustrated.

PRESSURE HALF TIME

- The pressure half time principle was adopted by echo from the 1968 cath paper by Libanoff and Rodbard, which provides elegant pressure figures.

Libanoff AJ, Rodbard S. Atrioventricular pressure half-time. Measure of mitral valve orifice area. Circulation. 1968;38:144–150. Full PDF: www.ahajournals.org/doi/pdf/10.1161/01.CIR.38.1.144

- Remember: Cath is good in measuring pressures but cannot measure blood flow velocities. Echo measures velocities and pressure gradients, but not actual pressures.

- Pressure half time principle: The time that it takes for the diastolic pressure across the mitral valve to drop by half is proportional to the mitral stenosis valve area—irrespective of heart rate. The worse the stenosis, the longer the half time.

- Translation: Pressure half time formula works in mitral stenosis patients even after they develop atrial fibrillation. It is fairly consistent from diastole to diastole, irrespective of cardiac cycle length. You can choose to use the longer cycles for technically easier measurements.

- Sample calculation of pressure half time in a mitral stenosis patient with a measured E *velocity* of 2 m/s:

  1. Go from velocities to pressures.

     $4V^2$ "takes you from velocities to pressures".

     "Pressure question" in this case would be:

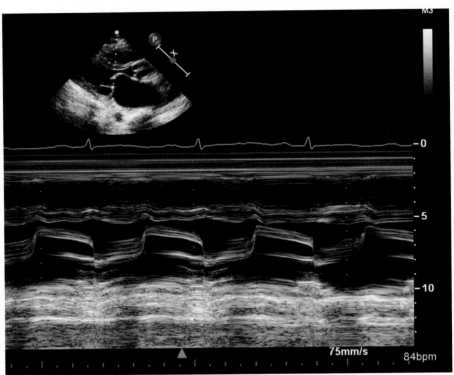

FIGURE 12-1. Mitral stenosis with a "hockey stick" anterior mitral leaflet on 2D (shown on the upper part of the image). M-mode beam passing through the anterior and posterior mitral leaflets shows the classic plateau of the anterior mitral leaflet EF slope. There is also a second, more subtle finding. The posterior mitral leaflet is being pulled anteriorly by the bigger anterior leaflet. This is due to the commissural fusion caused by inflammation during the initial episode of rheumatic fever.

- How long does it take for the pressure gradient to drop from 16 mm Hg ($4 \times 2 \times 2$) to 8 mm Hg?

2. Now that you calculated the target half time *pressure*, go back from pressures to velocities.

To go back to velocities:

- "UnBernoulli" the calculated 8 mm Hg pressure gradient in this patient back to a velocity:

a. Divide 8 by 4.

b. Calculate the square root:

$8 \div 4 = 2$; square root of 2 = 1.4 m/s.

Same question (now a "velocity question"):

- How long in milliseconds does it take for the original 2 m/s E velocity in this patient to drop to 1.4 m/s?

• This pressure half *time* in milliseconds is easily measured on the Doppler mitral inflow tracing in mitral stenosis. Do it yourself! Don't let the computer do it for you, or you will never learn to "cook the numbers on the fly" during a conversation about the severity of the stenosis (see examples below).

3. Calculate mitral stenosis area by dividing the accepted constant of 220 ms by the calculated pressure half time in this patient.

Formula: 220 ÷ calculated pressure half time = mitral stenosis area.

- Examples:
  - Severe mitral stenosis: A patient with a *long* calculated pressure half time of 440 ms has a valve area of 0.5 cm^2.
  - Mild mitral stenosis: A patient with a *short* calculated pressure half time of 110 ms has a valve area of 2.0 cm^2.
- Pressure half time pitfalls:
- In the case of a bimodal (initially steep) deceleration slope:
  - Use another slope if possible.
  - Do the calculation in mid-diastole rather than using the early deceleration slope.
- **Caution: *Associated conditions* can cause overestimation of mitral stenosis orifice area.**
  - Hemodynamically significant aortic regurgitation will *shorten* mitral pressure half time.
  - Elevated left ventricular end-diastolic pressure in an associated dilated cardiomyopathy will *shorten* mitral pressure half time.
  - Noncompliant hypertrophied hypertensive left ventricle will *shorten* mitral pressure half time.
- Note: The criteria for severe mitral stenosis were changed in the recent guidelines:
  - Resting mean pressure gradient ≥10 mm Hg.
  - Mitral valve area ≤1.5 cm^2.
  - Pressure half time ≥150 ms.

de Agustin JA, Mejia H, Viliani D, et al. **Proximal flow convergence** method by three-dimensional color Doppler echocardiography for mitral valve area assessment in rheumatic mitral stenosis. J Am Soc Echocardiogr. 2014;27:838–845.

Nunes MC, Tan TC, Elmariah S, et al. The **echo score** revisited: impact of incorporating commissural morphology and leaflet displacement to the prediction of outcome for patients undergoing percutaneous mitral valvuloplasty. Circulation. 2014;129:886–895.

Reis G, Motta MS, Barbosa MM, et al. **Dobutamine stress** echocardiography for noninvasive assessment and risk stratification of patients with rheumatic mitral stenosis. J Am Coll Cardiol. 2004;43:393–401.

Dobutamine stress echo is safe in patients with mitral stenosis. A mean gradient ≥18 mm Hg identifies a subgroup of high-risk patients.

Wunderlich NC, Beigel R, Siegel RJ. Management of mitral stenosis using 2D and 3D echo-Doppler **imaging**. JACC Cardiovasc Imaging. 2013;6:1191–1205.

OTHER MITRAL STENOSIS MEASUREMENT TECHNIQUES

- Planimetry
  - Reference mitral stenosis measurement—to which other measurement techniques are compared.

- Reliability is unaffected by ventricular function, loading conditions, or associated valve disorders.
- Technically challenging—requires patience and experience.
- The ultrasound beam must be perpendicular to the mitral leaflet tips in the short-axis view.
- The narrowest orifice is selected by scanning slowly from apex to base.
- 3D transthoracic and transesophageal imaging improves accuracy.

• Mean gradient
- Pressure gradient calculated from the mitral inflow velocity.
- Easily measured.
- Affected by heart rate and blood flow.
- May be significantly elevated in the absence of mitral stenosis.

• PISA
- Mitral volume flow is divided by the maximum velocity of mitral inflow.
- Calculation can be performed even with coexisting mitral regurgitation.

• Continuity
- Ratio between (right or left) ventricular outflow stroke volume and mitral inflow VTI.
- Concept: Flow is the same across the mitral, aortic, and pulmonic valves.
- Pitfall: Ventricular outflow and mitral annulus are wrongly assumed to be perfectly circular.
- Pitfall: Invalid with severe valvular regurgitation.

• Mitral valve resistance
- Ratio of mean mitral gradient to transmitral diastolic flow rate.
- Calculated by dividing stroke volume by diastolic filling period.
- Argued to be less dependent on flow conditions.
- Correlates with pulmonary artery pressure.

Dreyfus J, Brochet E, Lepage L, et al. Real-time 3D **transesophageal** measurement of the mitral valve area in patients with mitral stenosis. Eur J Echocardiogr. 2011;12:750–755.

Faletra F, Pezzano A Jr, Fusco R, et al. Measurement of mitral valve area in mitral stenosis: four **echocardiographic methods** compared with direct measurement of anatomic orifices. J Am Coll Cardiol. 1996;28:1190–1197.

Izgi C, Ozdemir N, Cevik C, et al. Mitral valve resistance as a determinant of resting and stress pulmonary artery pressure in patients with mitral stenosis: a dobutamine stress study. J Am Soc Echocardiogr. 2007;20:1160–1166.

Rifkin RD, Harper K, Tighe D. Comparison of proximal **isovelocity surface area** method with pressure half-time and planimetry in evaluation of mitral stenosis. J Am Coll Cardiol. 1995;26:458–465.

Zamorano J, Cordeiro P, Sugeng L, et al. Real-time **three-dimensional** echocardiography for rheumatic mitral valve stenosis evaluation: an accurate and novel approach. J Am Coll Cardiol. 2004;43:2091–2096.

MITRAL STENOSIS SCANNING TIPS

• $0.29 \times$ deceleration time = pressure half time (Fig. 12-2).
• Planimetry of a funnel-shaped rheumatic mitral stenosis orifice is typically performed at a subvalvular plane.

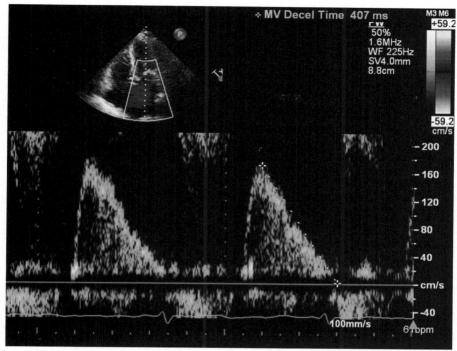

FIGURE 12-2. 0.29 × deceleration time = pressure half time.

- Older, hypertrophied, or failing left ventricles may shorten pressure half time in mitral stenosis.
- Older, hypertrophied left ventricles with impaired relaxation may have a prolonged pressure half time. If there is no mitral stenosis, the E velocity is not increased (<1 m/s).
- Mean gradient in severe mitral stenosis may be low when echo shows decreased cardiac output.
- Atrial fibrillation is common in mitral stenosis. Wait for a long cardiac cycle to measure the pressure half time. Measure multiple cycles for consistency.
- Always report the heart rate at which pressure half time was measured.
- Remember to look for pulmonary hypertension—it affects dyspnea and exercise tolerance in mitral stenosis.
- Learn the echocardiographic scoring for possible balloon valvotomy: leaflet mobility, leaflet thickening, leaflet calcification, subvalvular involvement.
- Mitral valves with heavy calcification, chordal shortening, fibrosis, and extensive subvalvular involvement are less amenable to balloon valvotomy.
- Global longitudinal strain is a powerful predictor of long-term outcome after successful valvotomy.
- An elevated mean gradient after valvotomy indicates unresolved elevated left atrial pressure.

*Abascal VM, Wilkins GT, Choong CY, et al. Echocardiographic evaluation of mitral valve structure and function in patients followed for at least 6 months after percutaneous balloon mitral **valvuloplasty**. J Am Coll Cardiol. 1988;12:606–615.*

*Barros-Gomes S, Eleid MF, Dahl JS, et al. Predicting outcomes after percutaneous mitral balloon valvotomy: the impact of left ventricular **strain** imaging. Eur Heart J Cardiovasc Imaging. 2017;18:763–771.*

*Cannan CR, Nishimura RA, Reeder GS, et al. Echocardiographic assessment of **commissural calcium**: a simple predictor of outcome after percutaneous mitral balloon valvotomy. J Am Coll Cardiol. 1997;29:175–180.*

Inoue K, Owaki T, Nakamura T, et al. Clinical application of transvenous mitral commissurotomy by a new balloon catheter. J Thorac Cardiovasc Surg. 1984;87:394–402.

Iung B, Cormier B, Ducimetiere P, et al. Functional results 5 years after successful percutaneous mitral commissurotomy in a series of 528 patients and analysis of predictive factors. J Am Coll Cardiol. 1996;27:407–414.

Song JK, Kang DH, Lee CW, et al. Factors determining the exercise capacity in mitral stenosis. Am J Cardiol. 1996;78: 1060–1062.

Wilkins GT, Weyman AE, Abascal VM, et al. Percutaneous balloon dilatation of the mitral valve: an analysis of echocardiographic variables related to outcome and the mechanism of dilatation. Br Heart J. 1988;60:299–308.

MITRAL ANNULAR CALCIFICATION

- Mitral annular calcification (MAC) is a common finding in the elderly.
- It is also found in younger patients with end-stage renal disease. MAC may predispose the mitral valve to infection with endocarditis in this population.
- MAC typically involves the posterior mitral leaflet annulus where it joins the left ventricular wall (Fig. 12-3).

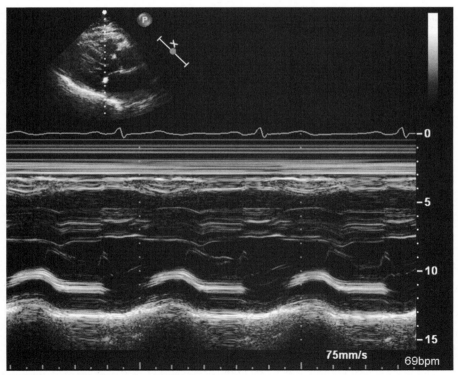

FIGURE 12-3. Mitral annular calcification.

- A rare *caseous* variant may be manifested on the echocardiogram as calcification with an echolucent center. The appearance may suggest endocarditis with an abscess; the mitral valve must be carefully scrutinized for vegetations or leaflet perforation.
- The extent of calcification does not correlate with the degree of mitral valve obstruction.
- Planimetry of the mitral area may not be possible when there are excessive artifacts from the calcium.
- Doppler is required (to determine whether suspected valvular stenosis is really present) when leaflet mobility is unclear on 2D echo images.
- There are *pitfalls* in the echocardiographic interpretation of associated findings.
- There is a tendency to overdiagnose mitral stenosis in patients with MAC:
  - Pressure half time may be clinically misleading (suggesting stenosis) if done with continuous-wave Doppler. The isovolumic relaxation time will not be prolonged in valvular stenosis.
  - The presence of MAC affects the velocity of adjacent myocardium. Tissue Doppler interpretation of diastolic and systolic LV function also may be misleading.
  - The left atrium may be enlarged due to age, diastolic dysfunction, or associated mitral regurgitation. Left atrial enlargement does not diagnose calcific mitral stenosis in patients with MAC.
- However, calcific extension to the mitral valve in patients with aortic stenosis has been shown to cause significant non-rheumatic mitral stenosis.

Carpentier AF, Pellerin M, Fuzellier JF, et al. Extensive calcification of the mitral valve anulus: pathology and surgical management. J Thorac Cardiovasc Surg. 1996;111:718–729.

Extensive expert **surgical paper**. Complete annulus decalcification and valve repair can be done safely in patients with mitral valve regurgitation, even when the calcification process deeply involves the myocardium.

Deluca G, Correale M, Ieva R, et al. The incidence and clinical course of **caseous** calcification of the mitral annulus: a prospective echocardiographic study. J Am Soc Echocardiogr. 2008;21:828–833.

- *An active, changing process, where caseous necrosis of a mix of calcium, cholesterol, and fatty acids appears on echo as a large posterior mitral annular calcification.*
- *The borders are smooth, and the center is somewhat more echolucent.*
- *It is not a tumor, an abscess, or a vegetation.*
- *A different histologic composition has been described with the same echocardiographic appearance (amorphous eosinophilic acellular material surrounded by macrophages and lymphocytes).*

Iwataki M, Takeuchi M, Otani K, et al. **Calcific extension** towards the mitral valve causes non-rheumatic mitral stenosis in degenerative aortic stenosis: real-time 3D transoesophageal echocardiography study. Open Heart. 2014;1:e000136.

Pomerance A. **Pathological** and clinical study of calcification of the mitral valve ring. J Clin Pathol. 1970;23:354–361.

PARACHUTE MITRAL VALVE AND MITRAL ARCADE

- *Parachute* mitral valve is a rare congenital disorder of the mitral valve that can cause mitral stenosis:
  - There is obstruction to mitral inflow at the level of the chordae.
  - The mitral chordae insert into a single papillary muscle.
  - The preferential insertion is difficult to prove with long-axis 2D echo views.
  - Short-axis views can show deviation of the mitral opening toward a preferred papillary muscle (typically the posteromedial).
- Mitral *arcade* is another rare abnormality created by thickening and shortening of the mitral leaflet chordae.
- Scanning tip: Always make a mental note of the chordal distance from the papillary muscle tips to the mitral leaflet body.

Hakim FA, Krishnaswamy C, Mookadam F. Mitral arcade in adults—a systematic **overview**. Echocardiography. 2013;30: 354–359.

Kutty S, Cohen TM, Smallhorn JF. **Three-dimensional** echocardiography in the assessment of congenital mitral valve disease. J Am Soc Echocardiogr. 2014;27:142–154.

Mohan JC, Shukla M, Mohan V, et al. **Spectrum** of congenital mitral valve abnormalities associated with solitary undifferentiated papillary muscle in adults. Indian Heart J. 2016;68:639–645.

Oosthoek PW, Wenink AC, Wisse LJ, et al. **Development** of the papillary muscles of the mitral valve: morphogenetic background of parachute-like asymmetric mitral valves and other mitral valve anomalies. J Thorac Cardiovasc Surg. 1998;116:36–46.

Séguéla PE, Houyel L, Acar P. Congenital **malformations** of the mitral valve. Arch Cardiovasc Dis. 2011;104:465–479.

Sormani P, Chiara B, Taglieri C, et al. Echocardiographic **assessment** and successful valvular repair of congenital mitral arcade. J Cardiovasc Echogr. 2015;25:57–59.

LUTEMBACHER SYNDROME

- Lutembacher syndrome is a previously rare cardiac abnormality characterized by the combination of an atrial septal defect with mitral stenosis.
- Correct diagnosis is important. It prompts appropriate treatment by percutaneous transcatheter intervention.
- The pathophysiology is important to recognize in the current era. The number of cardiac patients undergoing procedures with transseptal puncture is increasing dramatically.
- Scanning note: The pressure half time method becomes an inaccurate measure of the stenotic mitral valve area when a depressurizing atrial shunt coexists with mitral stenosis. Planimetry and continuity equation methods have to be used to determine mitral stenosis valve area in Lutembacher syndrome.

Lutembacher R. De la stenose mitrale avec communication interauriculaire. Arch Mal Coeur. 1916;9:237–260.

Ngu KB, Sliwa K, Kengne AP. et al. Current diagnostic and treatment strategies for Lutembacher syndrome: the pivotal role of echocardiography. Cardiovasc Diagn Ther. 2015;5:122–132.

Tezcan M, Isilak Z, Atalay M, et al. Echocardiographic assessment of Lutembacher syndrome. Kardiol Pol. 2014;72:660.

Vasan RS, Shrivastava S, Kumar MV. Value and limitations of Doppler echocardiographic determination of mitral valve area in Lutembacher syndrome. J Am Coll Cardiol. 1992;20:1362–1370.

VIDEOS

VIDEO 12-1 (A–H). Mitral leaflet doming in mitral stenosis.

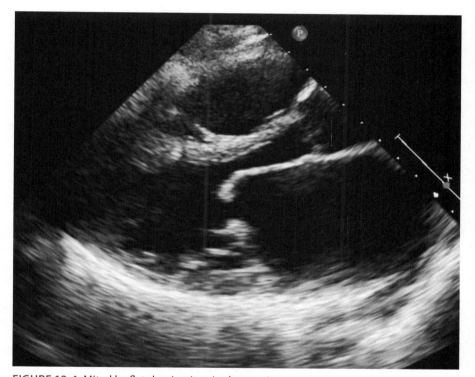

FIGURE 12-4. Mitral leaflet doming in mitral stenosis.

VIDEO 12-2. Short-axis view of a stenotic mitral orifice.

VIDEO 12-3. Mitral stenosis steep and flat slopes. Pressure half time is measured using the flatter slope.

VIDEO 12-4. Thick mitral valve chordae.

VIDEO 12-5 (A–C). Balloon valvuloplasty for mitral stenosis.

VIDEO 12-6. Mitral leaflet calcification indicates that the apical tethering is not acute.

VIDEO 12-7. Mitral chordae that attach to the body of the leaflet (not the commissure) are called secondary chordae.

VIDEO 12-8. Apical tethering of the posterior mitral leaflet with calcification of the posterior mitral leaflet.

VIDEO 12-9 (A–C). Double-orifice clipped mitral valve.

VIDEO 12-10. 3D guidance of MitraClip insertion.

VIDEO 12-11. Mirror artifact of the mitral valve.

VIDEO 12-12. Mitral annular calcification.

VIDEO 12-13. Mitral annular calcification. Attenuation artifact.

VIDEO 12-14 (A,B). Attenuation artifact from mitral annular calcium partly masking the coronary sinus.

VIDEO 12-15 (A–E). Caseous calcification of the mitral annulus.

CHAPTER 13

Prosthetic Valves

GUIDELINES

Zoghbi WA, Chambers JB, Dumesnil JG, et al. Recommendations for evaluation of prosthetic valves with echocardiography and Doppler ultrasound. J Am Soc Echocardiogr. 2009;22:975–1014.

- Side-by-side images in this document illustrate normal and abnormal prosthesis function.
- Tables 13-1 and 13-2 provide parameters for mild and severe prosthesis malfunction.
- There are echo parameters for comprehensive evaluation.

*Lancellotti P, Pibarot P, Chambers J, et al. Recommendations for the **imaging** assessment of prosthetic heart valves. Eur Heart J Cardiovasc Imaging. 2016;17:589–590.*

- This is an extensive document that covers all topics related to prosthetic valves.
- The digital version should be downloaded and used for reference.

*Rosenhek R, Binder T, Maurer G, Baumgartner H. **Normal values** for Doppler echocardiographic assessment of heart valve prostheses. J Am Soc Echocardiogr. 2003;16:1116–1127.*

DOPPLER EVALUATION OF PROSTHETIC AORTIC VALVES

- The simplified Bernoulli equation is used for gradients.
- The gradient of prosthetic aortic valves may be *overestimated* by this method if:
  - Cardiac output is increased.
  - Left ventricular outflow is narrow.
  - Prosthesis ring size is small.
  - Proximal ascending aorta is small.
- For continuity calculations of aortic prosthesis area:
  - It is necessary to measure the outflow diameter directly.

TABLE 13-1 • Normal vs. Stenotic Prosthesis

Aortic Prosthesis	Normal	Stenotic
Peak velocity	<3 m/s	>4 m/s
Mean gradient	<20 mm Hg	>35 mm Hg
Doppler velocity index	>0.30	<0.25
Effective orifice area	>1.2 cm²	<0.8 cm²
Jet velocity contour	Triangular	Rounded
Acceleration time	<80 ms	>100 ms

Note: Peak velocity and mean gradient are affected by increased systolic blood flow if there is an increase in stroke volume due to coexisting aortic prosthesis regurgitation.

- The label size of the prosthesis should not be used as a substitute.
- The Doppler velocity index (DVI) is a simplification:
  - It is the ratio of the velocity *proximal to* the valve and the velocity *through* the valve.

Bach DS. Echo/Doppler evaluation of hemodynamics after aortic valve replacement: principles of interrogation and evaluation of **high gradients**. JACC Cardiovasc Imaging. 2010;3:296–304. See Table 13-1.

PROSTHESIS BACKWASH

- Prosthetic mechanical valves are intentionally designed to have small leaks by two mechanisms:
  - Closure backflow: A certain amount of blood flow reversal is required to close the valve. Closure backflow *stops* once the occluder mechanism is properly seated in the sewing ring.
  - Leakage backflow: This is a predesigned small amount of retrograde flow that *continues* after the occluder is properly seated and should not be interpreted as prosthesis malfunction.

PRESSURE RECOVERY

- Pressure recovery offers an explanation for a higher Doppler gradient and lower catheterization gradient across a bileaflet aortic prosthetic valve.
- The explanation:
  - Kinetic energy is recovered in the form of a pressure rise/recovery as blood crosses a prosthetic aortic valve.
  - A catheter "catches" the rising pressure in the aorta.
  - The same catheter misses a high localized gradient right past the valve because it is *distal* to that location. Remember that catheters measure pressures, not pressure gradients.
  - Careful Doppler interrogation can find this high localized gradient.
- Result: Doppler gradient is higher. Catheter gradient is lower.

Vandervoort PM, Greenberg NL, Powell KA, et al. Pressure recovery in bileaflet heart valve prostheses. Localized high velocities and gradients in central and side orifices with implications for Doppler-catheter gradient relation in aortic and mitral position. Circulation. 1995;92:3464–3472.

PROSTHESIS–PATIENT MISMATCH

- This is an abnormally high prosthesis gradient because it is too small for a patient's body size.
- It is important to calculate *indexed* aortic valve area.
- If the projected postoperative indexed aortic valve area is anticipated to be too small, the aortic root may need to be enlarged, and an alternate prosthesis may be necessary.

PANNUS

Long-term progressive deposition of fibrous tissue on prosthetic leaflets.

- Hemodynamic problems (regurgitation and/or stenosis) caused by pannus deposition are chronic and progressive.
- Acute onset of regurgitation or stenosis suggests *thrombus* rather than pannus.

Scanning note: It is important to distinguish the echocardiographic signs of severe versus the signs of mild mitral prosthesis regurgitation (Table 13-2).

HEMOLYTIC ANEMIA

- May occur when there is rapid acceleration and deceleration of blood flow near a prosthetic mitral valve.
- Abnormal lab tests indicating hemolysis:
  - Severe anemia.
  - Increased reticulocyte count.
  - Decreased haptoglobin.
  - Increased LDH.
- The anemia is discovered an average of 3 months after the surgery.

TABLE 13-2 • Mitral Prosthesis Regurgitation		
Mitral Prosthesis Regurgitation	**Mild**	**Severe**
Left ventricular dimensions	Normal	Dilated
TEE appearance	Normal	Abnormal
Color flow jet area	<4 cm^2	>8 cm^2
Percent of LA area	<20%	>40%
Flow convergence	Minimal	Large
CW jet density	Faint	Dense
CW jet contour	Rounded	Triangular
Pulmonary vein flow	Systolic dominant	Diastolic dominant and/or systolic flow reversal
Vena contracta (cm)	<0.3	≥0.6
Regurgitant volume (cc)	<30	≥60
Regurgitant fraction (%)	<30	≥50
Regurgitant orifice area (cm^2)	<0.2	≥0.50

Garcia MJ, Vandervoort P, Stewart WJ, et al. Mechanisms of hemolysis with mitral prosthetic regurgitation. Study using transesophageal echocardiography and fluid dynamic simulation. J Am Coll Cardiol. 1996;27:399–406.

- *Distinct **patterns of regurgitant flow** are seen in patients with mitral prosthetic hemolysis.*
- *They are associated with rapid acceleration and deceleration or high peak shear rates, or both.*
- *The nature of the flow disturbance produced by the prosthetic regurgitant lesion and the resultant increase in shear stress are more important than the site of origin of the flow disturbance in producing clinical hemolysis.*

Yeo TC, Freeman WK, Schaff HV, et al. **Mechanisms** of hemolysis after mitral valve repair: assessment by serial echocardiography. J Am Coll Cardiol. 1998;32:717–723.

Three mechanisms:

- *Direct **collision** of a mitral regurgitation jet with the surface of the annuloplasty ring.*
- *Dehiscence of an annuloplasty ring **fragmenting** the regurgitation jet.*
- *Rapid **acceleration** of the regurgitation jet in a small dehiscence.*

ROSS PROCEDURE

- The patient's own pulmonic valve is moved to the aortic position (called a neo-aortic valve or an autograft valve).
- A donor (homograft) pulmonic valve is put in its place in the pulmonic position.

Savoye C, Auffray JL, Hubert E, et al. Echocardiographic follow-up after Ross procedure in 100 patients. Am J Cardiol. 2000;85:854–857.

- *There was 1 case of mild homograft regurgitation and 4 of mild autograft regurgitation at late follow-up.*
- *Autograft peak gradients were low and reproducible (5 ± 2.8 mm Hg at discharge vs. 5.5 ± 3.5 mm Hg at last follow-up; p = NS).*
- *Homograft **peak gradients increased significantly** without severe obstruction (7.8 ± 5.7 mm Hg at discharge vs. 15.8 ± 9.2 mm Hg at last follow-up). The diameter of the autograft annulus was stable during follow-up, whereas autograft dimensions at sinuses and proximal aorta increased significantly. For 10% of patients, there was a 20% dilation of sinus diameters, but in only 3 patients (3%) was this beyond the upper normal limit.*

PROSTHETIC VALVES IN PEDIATRICS

- Some pediatric prosthetic valves are placed in a supra-annular position.
- The Ross procedure is performed in some children with aortic stenosis.
- There may be a *conduit* in the pulmonary artery in pediatric patients with:
  - Rastelli repair for transposition with outflow obstruction.
  - Neonatal repair of tetralogy with pulmonary atresia.
  - Yasui procedure for interrupted aortic arch.
  - Sano revision of hypoplastic left heart syndrome.
- Technical point: Tricuspid regurgitation velocity should be correlated with conduit gradients.

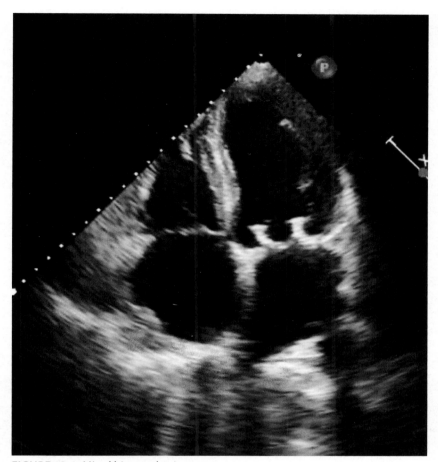

FIGURE 13-1. Mitral bioprosthesis struts.

SCANNING TIPS

- Both the size and type of a prosthesis determine the Doppler velocities.
- The pressure half time method has not been validated for mitral and tricuspid prosthetic valves.
- It is thought that pressure half time overestimates the effective orifice area of mitral and tricuspid prosthetic valves.
- Transthoracic and transesophageal imaging are frequently combined to evaluate abnormal prosthetic valves.
- The effective orifice area of a prosthesis is significantly smaller than the prosthetic ring.
- Bioprosthetic mitral valves have three (not two) leaflets (Fig. 13-1).

(continued)

SCANNING TIPS (Continued)

- ■ Pericardial bioprosthetic valves may initially have a central regurgitant jet after implantation. The leaflets may have become rigid during the preservation process. After several weeks, this jet may decrease or disappear as the moving leaflets become more pliable.

- ■ Prosthetic valves in children who are growing may show worsening hemodynamics on serial echoes—stroke volume increases over time, while the valve orifice area remains unchanged.

- ■ A human aortic homograft (allograft) prosthesis is implanted in one of three ways:
    - Freehand valve implantation in the subcoronary position. (Search YouTube: *How to trim the aortic allograft*.)
    - Full root and valve replacement with coronary reimplantation.
    - Miniroot: implanted inside the native aortic root.

POSTOPERATIVE MOTION OF THE INTERVENTRICULAR SEPTUM

- The pericardium is usually left open after cardiac surgery.
- As a result, pericardial fluid is in communication with pleural fluid.

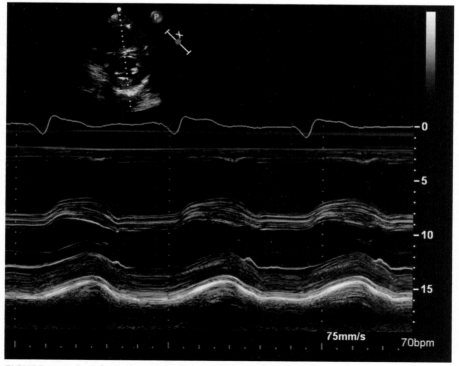

FIGURE 13-2. Paradoxical motion of the interventricular septum.

- This is done because there is less likelihood for postoperative tamponade, unless a thrombus forms in the pericardium.
- There is a typical associated M-mode abnormality of the interventricular septal motion due to resultant exaggerated anterior motion of the entire heart within the chest (Fig. 13-2).
- M-mode in the parasternal views shows:
  - Paradoxical motion of the interventricular septum.
  - Preserved systolic thickening of the abnormally displaced septum.
  - No brief initial downward deflection (unlike what is found in septal motion due to left bundle branch block).
- Pitfalls:
  - This finding makes wall motion analysis difficult.
  - It may vary with changes in cardiac volumes.
  - Coexisting bundle branch block, or right ventricular pressure/volume overload, may confound the interpretation of wall motion.
  - The finding may disappear several years after the surgery.

TAVR PROSTHESIS

- Transcatheter aortic valves need to be properly positioned before deployment.
- If the position is *too high*, there can be:
  - Coronary ostial occlusion.
  - Regurgitation.
  - Device embolization.
- If the position is *too low*, there can be:
  - Stent interference with mitral valve function.
  - Possible perforation of the anterior mitral leaflet.
  - Trauma to the cardiac conducting system.
- Post-TAVR transthoracic echo prior to discharge is used to:
  - Look for a new pericardial effusion.
  - Confirm proper device position.
  - Compare current to pre-existing mitral regurgitation.
  - Measure mean and maximum transcatheter gradients.
  - Calculate TAVR prosthesis effective orifice area by continuity.
  - Determine whether there is residual paravalvular TAVR regurgitation.

Alfonso F, Domínguez L, Rivero F, et al. Severe intraventricular **dynamic gradient** following transcatheter aortic valve implantation: suicide ventricle? EuroIntervention. 2015;11:e1

Gerckens U, Pizzulli L, Raisakis K. Alcohol septal ablation as a **bail-out** procedure for suicide left ventricle after transcatheter aortic valve implantation. J Invasive Cardiol. 2013;25:E114–E117.

Ibrahim H, Barker CM, Reardon MJ, et al. **Suicide left ventricle** due to conduction disturbance following transcatheter aortic valve replacement and reversal with restoration of sinus rhythm: is there life after death? J Invasive Cardiol. 2015;27:E107–E109.

Suh WM, Witzke CF, Palacios IF. Suicide left ventricle following transcatheter aortic valve implantation. Catheter Cardiovasc Interv. 2010;76:616–620.

Dynamic left ventricular outflow tract obstruction, and left ventricular mid-cavity obliteration, can complicate the TAVR postoperative course. Heart rate control, maintenance of sinus rhythm, pericardial fluid drainage, and intravascular fluid replacement may be lifesaving.

- In the case of residual paravalvular TAVR regurgitation:
  - Color-flow Doppler is used to look for multiple, possibly eccentric paravalvular regurgitation jets.
  - Color flow is used to map and measure the circumferential short-axis extent of paravalvular TAVR regurgitation.
  - Continuous-wave Doppler measures pressure half time of existing aortic regurgitation jets.
  - Doppler in the descending thoracic aorta looks for diastolic flow reversal.

Pislaru SV, Nkomo VT, Sandhu GS. **Assessment** of prosthetic valve function after TAVR. JACC Cardiovasc Imaging. 2016;9: 193–206.

Bloomfield GS, Gillam LD, Hahn RT, et al. A practical guide to **multimodality imaging** of transcatheter aortic valve replacement. JACC Cardiovasc Imaging. 2012;5:441–455.

Hahn RT, Kodali S, Tuzcu EM, et al. Echocardiographic imaging of **procedural complications** during balloon-expandable transcatheter aortic valve replacement. JACC Cardiovasc Imaging. 2015;8:288–318.

Comprehensive collection of images and online videos.

Otto CM, Kumbhani DJ, Alexander KP, et al. 2017 ACC Expert Consensus Decision Pathway for Transcatheter Aortic Valve Replacement. J Am Coll Cardiol. 2017;69:1313–1346.

Extensive practical checklists.

PROSTHETIC VALVE ENDOCARDITIS

- In patients with prosthetic valves:
  - Echo is performed for new fever associated with a changing or new murmur.
  - The more common causes of a fever should always be considered (respiratory tract or urinary tract infection).
  - Color-flow evidence of new paravalvular regurgitation in a previously normal prosthesis indicates suture dehiscence.
  - Suture dehiscence is suggestive of endocarditis, and also of a possible abscess.
  - Vegetations appear independently mobile and have low, rather than calcific, echogenicity—but it may not be possible to distinguish a vegetation from a thrombus.
  - Early after aortic valve replacement surgery, *edema* around the prosthetic ring may be hard to distinguish from an abscess.
  - Color flow may find a fistula.
  - TEE is necessary when TTE is negative. The procedures are complementary because of shadowing from the prosthesis.
  - When clinical suspicion for endocarditis is high but the echo is negative, it is acceptable to wait for 7–10 days and then repeat the echo.

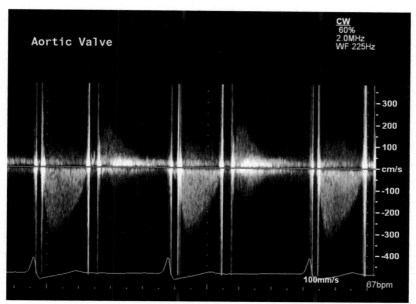

FIGURE 13-3. Filter saturation artifacts. Mitral and aortic prosthesis.

WALL FILTER SATURATION CROSSTALK ARTIFACTS

- Mechanical prosthetic valves create a short artifactual "spike" that can be used to determine timing of prosthetic leaflet opening and closing (Fig. 13-3).
- Continuous- and pulsed-wave Doppler interrogation of prosthetic mechanical leaflets overwhelms the Doppler filter circuits at the moment the leaflets open and close.
- This happens at the moment the ultrasound beam is perpendicular to the prosthesis leaflets. Strong momentary specular reflections return to the transducer and saturate the Doppler directional circuits. The dynamic range is excessive. The directional circuits cannot separate the signals properly. The wall filter does not work. A short artifact "spike" is generated. It marks the time of leaflet opening and closure on the Doppler display.
- This artifact can be put to good use. It is used to determine if prosthetic leaflets are sticking when they move.
- *Variable* leaflet opening and closing time intervals in a patient with a regular heart rhythm may provide indirect evidence of progressive pannus accumulation that may not be evident on 2D imaging of the valve.

Barbetseas J, Nagueh SF, Pitsavos C, et al. Differentiating thrombus from pannus formation in obstructed mechanical prosthetic valves: an evaluation of clinical, transthoracic and transesophageal echocardiographic parameters. J Am Coll Cardiol. 1998;32:1410–1417.

MITRAL PROSTHESIS SPEED ERROR

- The ultrasound system wrongly assumes that ultrasound propagates through a mechanical mitral valve at the speed of soft tissue.

- When scanning from the apical position, 2D mitral mechanical valve reflections may be displayed deeper than anatomically normal into the left atrium.

DOPPLER MIRROR ARTIFACT

- When interrogating the aortic arch with pulsed-wave Doppler, a weak signal may be displayed in the opposite direction of real flow.
- Decreasing the gain and changing the transducer angle helps to remove this artifact.
- Mirror artifacts can be created during color-flow Doppler evaluation of prosthetic mechanical mitral valves from the apical window:
  - Left ventricular outflow tract (LVOT) velocities reflect off the prosthesis.
  - The color-flow signal is "projected down" into the left atrium because of a longer transit time.
  - The resulting artifactual systolic color-flow pattern can resemble mitral regurgitation and may prompt an evaluation with TEE.
  - These mirror image LVOT artifacts in the left atrium can be identified by pulsed-wave interrogation of shape, velocity, and duration of the "relocated" LVOT Doppler signal, which will be different from a mitral regurgitation jet.

Linka AZ, Barton M, Attenhofer Jost C, et al. Doppler mirror image artifacts mimicking mitral regurgitation in patients with mechanical bileaflet mitral valve prostheses. Eur J Echocardiogr. 2000;1:138–143.

Rudski LG, Chow CM, Levine RA. Prosthetic mitral regurgitation can be mimicked by Doppler color flow mapping: avoiding misdiagnosis. J Am Soc Echocardiogr. 2004;17:829–833.

LEFT ATRIAL DISSECTION

- This is a rare disorder.
- It can occur spontaneously or after mitral valve surgery.
- Other causes:
  - Thoracic trauma.
  - Myocardial infarction.
  - Endocarditis.

*Choi JH, Kang JK, Park KJ, et al. Images in cardiovascular medicine. **Spontaneous** left atrial dissection presenting as pulmonary edema. Circulation. 2005;111:e372–373.*

*Cordero Lorenzana ML, López Pérez JM, Merayo Macías E, et al. Left atrial dissection and infective **endocarditis**. Rev Esp Cardiol. 1998;51:402–403.*

*Gallego P, Oliver JM, González A, et al. Left atrial dissection: pathogenesis, clinical course, and transesophageal **echocardiographic recognition**. J Am Soc Echocardiogr. 2001;14:813–820.*

*Jani S, Hecht S, Leibowitz K, et al. Left atrial dissection: an unusual complication of **mitral valve surgery**. Echocardiography. 2007;24:443–444.*

*Lombardo A, Luciani N, Rizzello V, et al. Images in cardiovascular medicine. Spontaneous left atrial dissection and hematoma **mimicking a cardiac tumor**: findings from echocardiography, cardiac computed tomography, magnetic resonance imaging, and pathology. Circulation. 2006;114:e249–250.*

*Martinez-Sellés M, García-Fernandez MA, Moreno M, et al. **Echocardiographic features** of left atrial dissection. Eur J Echocardiogr. 2000;1:147–150.*

VIDEOS

VIDEO 13-1 (A–C). Paravalvular aortic prosthesis regurgitation.

VIDEO 13-2. Mirror-image artifact from an aortic prosthesis.

VIDEO 13-3. Venetian blind reverberation artifact. Presumed reverberation from valve surface to transducer surface. Aortic prosthesis.

VIDEO 13-4. Comet tail presumed internal intraleaflet reverberation artifact. Mechanical aortic prosthesis.

VIDEO 13-5. Arc-shaped sidelobe artifact. Mechanical aortic prosthesis.

VIDEO 13-6. Arc-shaped sidelobe artifact and comet tail reverberation artifact. Mechanical aortic prosthesis.

VIDEO 13-7 (A,B). Reverberation and attenuation artifacts from a TAVR prosthesis.

VIDEO 13-8. TAVR prosthesis regurgitation.

VIDEO 13-9 (A,B). Aortic prosthesis. Sinus of Valsalva aneurysm.

VIDEO 13-10 (A,B). Prosthetic mitral ring.

VIDEO 13-11. Reverberation artifact from a prosthetic mitral ring.

VIDEO 13-12. Arc-shaped artifact. Mechanical prosthetic mitral valve. Respiratory "bounce" of the interventricular septum.

VIDEO 13-13. Aortic prosthesis endocarditis. Rocking due to partial ring dehiscence.

VIDEO 13-14 (A–C). Partial dehiscence of a prosthetic mitral ring.

VIDEO 13-15. Partial dehiscence of a mechanical mitral prosthesis.

VIDEO 13-16. Mitral bioprosthesis suture thread dehiscence.

VIDEO 13-17. Mitral bioprosthesis. Mild leaflet thickening.

VIDEO 13-18. Loose chordae (not vegetations) after chordal-sparing mitral bioprosthesis implant.

VIDEO 13-19 (A–C). Mitral mechanical bileaflet prosthesis.

VIDEO 13-20. Cavitation caused by a mitral mechanical bileaflet prosthesis.

VIDEO 13-21. Intermittent sticking of a mitral prosthesis leaflet.

VIDEO 13-22. Mitral bileaflet prosthesis. Dense spontaneous contrast ("smoke") in the left atrial appendage.

VIDEO 13-23 (A,B). Thrombus on the atrial side of a mitral prosthesis.

VIDEO 13-24. Reverberation artifact from a prosthetic mechanical aortic valve.

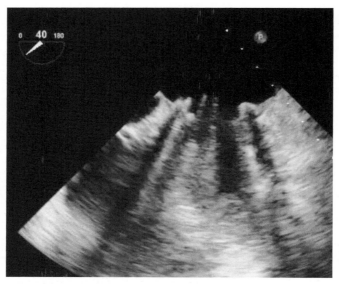

FIGURE 13-4. Comet tail reverberation artifact from a mechanical bileaflet mitral valve.

VIDEO 13-25. Mitral bioprosthetic valves have three leaflets.

VIDEO 13-26. Thick mitral bioprosthesis leaflets.

VIDEO 13-27. Mitral bioprosthesis. Puff-like pulmonary vein inflow into the left atrium. Tricuspid regurgitation.

VIDEO 13-28. Mitral bioprosthesis. Chordal sparing.

VIDEO 13-29. Mitral prosthetic ring.

VIDEO 13-30. Tricuspid bioprosthesis.

VIDEO 13-31. Mild tricuspid bioprosthesis regurgitation.

VIDEO 13-32 (A,B). Speed error artifact from a tricuspid prosthesis.

VIDEO 13-33 (A–C). Speed error artifact from a mitral prosthesis.

VIDEO 13-34. Cavitation artifact and speed error artifact from a mitral prosthesis.

VIDEO 13-35 (A–C). Aortic bioprosthesis.

VIDEO 13-36. Decreased aortic bioprosthesis leaflet excursion due to decreased left ventricular stroke volume.

VIDEO 13-37 (A,B). Starr Edwards ball-in-cage prosthesis—color "horns."

VIDEO 13-38. Fluoroscopy of a Starr Edwards prosthesis.

VIDEO 13-39 (A,B). Ultrasound scatter and range ambiguity artifacts caused by a breast implant.

- In our example:

  196 + 15 = 211

  211 − 120 = LVOT gradient

Note: Amyl nitrite inhalation may be administered to provoke a gradient during imaging with continuous wave Doppler.

Marwick TH, Nakatani S, Haluska B, et al. Provocation of latent left ventricular outflow tract gradients with **amyl nitrite** and exercise in hypertrophic cardiomyopathy. Am J Cardiol. 1995;75:805–809.

Zemanek D, Tomasov P, Homolova S, et al. Sublingual **isosorbide** dinitrate for the detection of obstruction in hypertrophic cardiomyopathy. Eur J Echocardiogr. 2011;12:684–687.

SYSTOLIC ANTERIOR MOTION

"Sharp anterior and superior angulation of the anterior mitral valve leaflet due to drag forces."

- Variable degree of contact of the anterior mitral leaflet to the septum in early to mid systole.
- M-mode categories:
  - Mild: SAM–septal distance of >10 mm.
  - Moderate: SAM–septal distance of 10 mm or less, or brief mitral leaflet–septal contact (<30% of echocardiographic systole).
  - Severe: Prolonged SAM–septal contact, lasting for at least 30% of echocardiographic systole.

Jiang L, Levine RA, King ME, Weyman AE. An integrated **mechanism** for systolic anterior motion of the mitral valve in hypertrophic cardiomyopathy based on echocardiographic observations. Am Heart J. 1987;113:633–644.

Kaple RK, Murphy RT, DiPaola LM, et al. **Mitral valve abnormalities** in hypertrophic cardiomyopathy: echocardiographic features and surgical outcomes. Ann Thorac Surg. 2008;85:1527–1535.

Sherrid MV, Chu CK, Delia E, et al. An echocardiographic study of the fluid **mechanics of obstruction** in hypertrophic cardiomyopathy. J Am Coll Cardiol. 1993;22:816–825.

SCANNING TIPS

- A tangential oblique cut may falsely overestimate wall thickness.
- A moderator band may be erroneously added to the septal thickness measurement.
- Localized lateral wall hypertrophy may be missed in a standard parasternal view.
- Foreshortened apical views may miss apical hypertrophy.
- Contrast, harmonics, and focus adjustment help to diagnose apical hypertrophy.
- 3D can help define mitral leaflet elongation in hypertrophic cardiomyopathy.
- Left atrial enlargement is related to disease severity.
- An intracavitary gradient can be created during stress echo even in the absence of hypertrophic cardiomyopathy.

Zywica K, Jenni R, Pellikka PA, et al. Dynamic left ventricular outflow tract obstruction evoked by exercise echocardiography: prevalence and predictive factors in a prospective study. Eur J Echocardiogr. 2008;9:665–671.

Dawn B, Paliwal VS, Raza ST, et al. Left ventricular outflow tract obstruction provoked during dobutamine stress echocardiography predicts future chest pain, syncope, and near syncope. Am Heart J. 2005;149:908–916.

Paraskevaidis IA, Panou F, Papadopoulos C, et al. Evaluation of left atrial longitudinal function in patients with hypertrophic cardiomyopathy: a tissue Doppler imaging and two-dimensional strain study. Heart. 2009;95:483–489.

Woo A, Jedrzkiewicz S. The mitral valve in hypertrophic cardiomyopathy: it's a long story. Circulation. 2011;124:9–12.

Yang H, Woo A, Monakier D, et al. Enlarged left atrial volume in hypertrophic cardiomyopathy: a marker for disease severity. J Am Soc Echocardiogr. 2005;18:1074–1082.

STRAIN AND MYOCARDIAL TORSION

From the vantage point of the apex:

- The base of the normal heart rotates clockwise.
- The apex normally rotates counterclockwise, creating a wringing motion that stores energy.
- In hypertrophic cardiomyopathy, midventricular twist differs from normal and untwisting (diastolic suction) is delayed.
- Diastolic apical pressure may contribute to the development of an apical aneurysm, even in the absence of coronary artery disease.
- Color and pulsed-wave Doppler may demonstrate intracavitary left ventricular flow during isovolumic relaxation. This isovolumic flow may be base to apex, or apex to base.
- The velocities of isovolumic base-to-apex flow may be faster than the E velocity, which can lead to confusion.

Carasso S, Yang H, Woo A, et al. Diastolic myocardial mechanics in hypertrophic cardiomyopathy. J Am Soc Echocardiogr. 2010;23:164–171.

Carasso S, Yang H, Woo A, et al. Systolic myocardial mechanics in hypertrophic cardiomyopathy: novel concepts and implications for clinical status. J Am Soc Echocardiogr. 2008;21:675–683.

Nakamura T, Matsubara K, Furukawa K, et al. Diastolic paradoxic jet flow in patients with hypertrophic cardiomyopathy: evidence of concealed apical asynergy with cavity obliteration. J Am Coll Cardiol. 1992;19:516–524.

TISSUE DOPPLER IN SCREENING FOR HYPERTROPHIC CARDIOMYOPATHY

- Myocardial contraction and relaxation velocities, detected by tissue Doppler, are reduced in familial hypertrophic cardiomyopathy, including in those without evident hypertrophy on 2D imaging.

Gandjbakhch E, Gackowski A, Tezenas du Montcel S, et al. Early identification of mutation carriers in familial hypertrophic cardiomyopathy by combined echocardiography and tissue Doppler imaging. Eur Heart J. 2010;31: 1599–1607.

Nagueh SF, Bachinski LL, Meyer D, et al. Tissue Doppler imaging consistently detects myocardial abnormalities in patients with hypertrophic cardiomyopathy and provides a novel means for an early diagnosis before and independently of hypertrophy. Circulation. 2001;104:128–130.

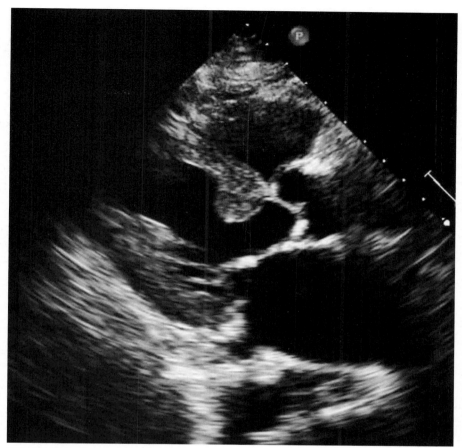

FIGURE 14-5. Sigmoid septum.

BASAL SEPTAL HYPERTROPHY IN THE ELDERLY

- Sigmoid septum, septal bulge, septal knuckle, discrete upper septal hypertrophy—all refer to the same echocardiographic finding.
- It may be an age-related finding associated with progressive angulation of the aorta.
- It may be either a subtype of HCM or a benign anatomic variant.
- Findings that are more compatible with a septal bulge rather than HCM of the elderly:
  - Focal hypertrophy.
  - Less than a 3 cm length of the basal anterior septum.
  - Protrusion of the focal hypertrophy into the LVOT (Fig. 14-5).
  - Normal LV end-diastolic diameter.
  - Absence of other echocardiographic findings of HCM.

Canepa M, Malti O, David M, et al. Prevalence, clinical correlates, and functional impact of subaortic ventricular septal bulge (from the Baltimore Longitudinal Study of Aging). Am J Cardiol. 2014;114:796–802.

Canepa M, Pozios I, Vianello PF, et al. Distinguishing ventricular septal bulge versus hypertrophic cardiomyopathy in the elderly. Heart. 2016;102:1087–1094.

Dalldorf FG, Willis PW. Angled aorta ("sigmoid septum") as a cause of hypertrophic stenosis. Hum Pathol. 1985;16:457–462.

Krasnow N. Subaortic septal bulge simulates hypertrophic cardiomyopathy by angulation of the septum with age, independent of focal hypertrophy: an echocardiographic study. J Am Soc Echocardiogr. 1997;10:545–555.

HYPERTROPHY IN THE ATHLETE

2015 Recommendations

Maron BJ, Udelson JE, Bonow RO, et al. Eligibility and Disqualification Recommendations for Competitive Athletes With Cardiovascular Abnormalities: Task Force 3: **Hypertrophic cardiomyopathy**, arrhythmogenic right ventricular cardiomyopathy and other cardiomyopathies, and myocarditis. Circulation. 2015;132:e273–e280.

There is a separate article on valvular heart disease in the athlete: Circulation 2015;132:e292–e297.

- Cardiac abnormalities that can increase the risk of sudden death during competitive sports:
  - Hypertrophic cardiomyopathy.
  - Arrhythmogenic right ventricular cardiomyopathy.
  - Marfan syndrome with a dilated aorta.
  - Coronary artery abnormalities.
  - Dilated cardiomyopathy.
- Individuals who exercise regularly for long periods of time may develop left ventricular hypertrophy, raising the question of possible hypertrophic cardiomyopathy.
- Some endurance athletes remodel their right ventricle. The echocardiographic findings in these athletes may resemble arrhythmogenic right ventricular cardiomyopathy.
- Left ventricular cavity dimensions may be increased in elite long-distance runners, rowers, and cyclists.
- Inferior vena cava may become dilated in elite swimmers.
- *Asymmetric* hypertrophy is uncommon.
- Significant left atrial enlargement should not be present.
- Diastolic left ventricular filling should be normal—not indicative of elevated left atrial pressures.
- Left ventricular wall thickness should regress with deconditioning.
- Strain imaging can be useful.
- Scanning note: The combination of chamber dilatation with the bradycardia of athletic conditioning can give a false visual impression of decreased systolic left ventricular function. Stroke volume should always be calculated. Strain imaging should be performed.

Butz T, van Buuren F, Mellwig KP, et al. Two-dimensional **strain** analysis of the global and regional myocardial function for the differentiation of pathologic and physiologic left ventricular hypertrophy: a study in athletes and in patients with hypertrophic cardiomyopathy. Int J Cardiovasc Imaging. 2011;27:91–100.

D'Ascenzi F, Pelliccia A, Natali BM, et al. Increased **left atrial size** is associated with reduced atrial stiffness and preserved reservoir function in athlete's heart. Int J Cardiovasc Imaging. 2015;31:699–705.

de Gregorio C, Speranza G, Magliarditi A, et al. **Detraining**-related changes in left ventricular wall thickness and longitudinal strain in a young athlete likely to have hypertrophic cardiomyopathy. J Sports Sci Med. 2012;11:557–561.

Pelliccia A, Maron BJ, Culasso F, et al. Athlete's heart in **women**. Echocardiographic characterization of highly trained elite female athletes. JAMA. 1996;276:211–215.

Simsek Z, Hakan Tas M, Degirmenci H, et al. **Speckle tracking** echocardiographic analysis of left ventricular systolic and diastolic functions of young elite athletes with eccentric and concentric type of cardiac remodeling. Echocardiography. 2013;30:1202–1208.

SEPTAL ETHANOL ABLATION

- Selective injection of ethanol into a septal perforator branch of the left anterior descending artery.
- The aim is to create a *targeted infarction* of the hypertrophic obstructive septum.
- Echocardiography has been used for guidance during the procedure and for subsequent monitoring.

Faber L, Ziemssen P, Seggewiss H. Targeting percutaneous transluminal septal ablation for hypertrophic obstructive cardio-myopathy by intraprocedural **echocardiographic monitoring**. J Am Soc Echocardiogr. 2000;13:1074–1079.

Liebregts M, Faber L, Jensen MK, et al. **Outcomes** of alcohol septal ablation in younger patients with obstructive hypertrophic cardiomyopathy. JACC Cardiovasc Interv. 2017;10:1134–1143.

Mazur W, Nagueh SF, Lakkis NM, et al. **Regression** of left ventricular hypertrophy after nonsurgical septal reduction therapy for hypertrophic obstructive cardiomyopathy. Circulation. 2001;103:1492–1496.

Nagueh SF, Lakkis NM, He ZX, et al. Role of myocardial **contrast** echocardiography during nonsurgical septal reduction therapy for hypertrophic obstructive cardiomyopathy. J Am Coll Cardiol. 1998;32:225–229.

Yoerger DM, Picard MH, Palacios IF, et al. Time course of pressure **gradient response** after first alcohol septal ablation for obstructive hypertrophic cardiomyopathy. Am J Cardiol. 2006;97:1511–1514.

FABRY DISEASE

- This is a rare, treatable enzyme deficiency that involves the heart.
- Because it is rare, it can remain unrecognized and may get misdiagnosed as hypertrophic cardiomyopathy.
- Tissue Doppler of the mitral annulus may show reduced systolic myocardial contraction and abnormal diastolic relaxation. Strain may be abnormal in the inferolateral wall.
- The tissue Doppler abnormalities are detectable even before the development of LVH.
- On 2D imaging, the *endocardial border* of the left ventricle has a distinctive bright-to-dark binary appearance in some of these patients.

Cantor WJ, Butany J, Iwanochko M, et al. **Restrictive** cardiomyopathy secondary to Fabry's disease. Circulation. 1998;98:1457–1459.

Chimenti C, Ricci R, Pieroni M, et al. Cardiac variant of Fabry's disease **mimicking** hypertrophic cardiomyopathy. Cardio-logia. 1999;44:469–473.

Desnick RJ, Blieden LC, Sharp HL, et al. Cardiac **valvular** anomalies in Fabry disease. Clinical, morphologic, and biochem-ical studies. Circulation. 1976;54:818–825.

There may be mitral valve thickening.

Kim WS, Kim HS, Shin J, et al. Prevalence of Fabry disease in Korean men with left ventricular hypertrophy. J Korean Med Sci. 2019;34:e63.

*The study identified **three patients** (0.3%) with Fabry disease **among 988** unselected Korean men with LVH. Although the prevalence of Fabry disease was low, early treatment of Fabry disease can result in a good prognosis. Therefore, in men with unexplained LVH, differential diagnosis of Fabry disease should be considered.*

Krämer J, Niemann M, Liu D, et al. Two-dimensional **speckle tracking** as a non-invasive tool for identification of myocardial fibrosis in Fabry disease. Eur Heart J. 2013;34:1587–1596.

Pieroni M, Chimenti C, Ricci R, et al. Early detection of Fabry cardiomyopathy by **tissue Doppler** imaging. Circulation. 2003;107:1978–1984.

Tissue Doppler imaging can provide a preclinical diagnosis of Fabry cardiomyopathy, allowing early institution of enzyme replacement therapy.

Sachdev B, Takenaka T, Teraguchi H, et al. Prevalence of Anderson-Fabry disease in male patients with **late onset** hypertrophic cardiomyopathy. Circulation. 2002;105:1407–1411.

Diagnosis is made in the third or fourth decade of life.

VIDEOS

VIDEO 14-1 (A–F). Asymmetric septal hypertrophy.

VIDEO 14-2. Basal septal hypertrophy.

VIDEO 14-3 (A–D). Systolic anterior motion of the mitral valve.

VIDEO 14-4. Decreased mitral leaflet coaptation with the systolic anterior motion.

VIDEO 14-5. Normal mitral leaflet motion. No systolic anterior motion.

VIDEO 14-6 (A–F). Apical left ventricular hypertrophy.

VIDEO 14-7 (A–F). Apical left ventricular hypertrophy. Spade-shaped contrast left ventriculogram.

VIDEO 14-8. Left ventricular outflow obstruction with "depressurizing" mitral regurgitation.

VIDEO 14-9. Left ventricular hypertrophy with end-systolic cavity obliteration.

VIDEO 14-10 (A,B). Severe left ventricular hypertrophy.

VIDEO 14-11. Mid-ventricular hypertrophy.

VIDEO 14-12. The moderator band in this image can give a false impression of septal hypertrophy.

- **Bonus quiz: Match the three bright reflections to the following: Annular calcium, nodule of Arantius, tricuspid chordae.**

VIDEO 14-13 (A,B). The moderator band in this image is seen only intermittently and can give a false impression of septal hypertrophy.

VIDEO 14-14 (A–C). Speckled "ground glass" appearance of the interventricular septum suggests myocardial fibrosis.

VIDEO 14-15. Anterolateral and posteromedial papillary muscles.

VIDEO 14-16. Left ventricular hypertrophy in a dialysis patient.

VIDEO 14-17. Left ventricular hypertrophy. Normal right ventricular wall thickness.

VIDEO 14-18. Biventricular hypertrophy. Small pericardial effusion. Possible infiltrative cardiomyopathy. Extensive mitral annular calcification is more common in dialysis patients than in infiltrative cardiomyopathies.

VIDEO 14-19 (A–D). Left ventricular trabeculations.

VIDEO 14-20. Small left ventricular internal dimensions. Reverberation artifact from a right ventricular pacemaker wire.

VIDEO 14-21. Asymmetric septal hypertrophy and abnormal wall motion.

VIDEO 14-22 (A–C). Peri-infarct hypertrophy. Basal septal hypertrophy with adjacent mid-to-apical septal infarction.

VIDEO 14-23 (A,B). Sigmoid septum due to sharp angulation of the aorta in relation to the interventricular septum.

VIDEO 14-24. Increased endocardial brightness can be a sign of Fabry cardiomyopathy.

VIDEO 14-25. Endocardial edge enhancement and reverberation artifact at the basal ventricular septum.

CHAPTER 15

Cardiomyopathies

2014 CLASSIFICATION

Arbustini E, Narula N, Tavazzi L, et al. The MOGE(S) classification of cardiomyopathy for clinicians. J Am Coll Cardiol. 2014;64:304–318.

- This classification of cardiomyopathies takes genetic testing into account.
- Many cardiomyopathies are familial diseases, and you will be scanning family members with questions about echo.
- MOGE(S):
  - **M**orphofunctional phenotype.
  - **O**rgan involvement.
  - **G**enetic inheritance pattern
  - **E**tiology including genetic defect, or underlying disease.
  - Functional **S**tatus.

DILATED CARDIOMYOPATHIES

- Echo is the primary imaging modality to establish *presence* and *severity* of dilated cardiomyopathy.
- Once the diagnosis is established, echo continues to be a valuable resource that helps to guide treatment and helps to estimate prognosis.
- Left ventricular chamber size is increased *by definition* in dilated cardiomyopathy (Fig. 15-1).
- Left ventricular stroke volume is decreased.
- Doppler evaluation: It is possible to use Doppler VTI measurements to serially follow changes in LV stroke volume.
- Technique: Left ventricular outflow tract (LVOT) area multiplied by VTI equals stroke volume. The LVOT area is assumed to remain unchanged from study to study.
- Therefore, Doppler VTI measurements alone can represent changes in LV stroke volume.

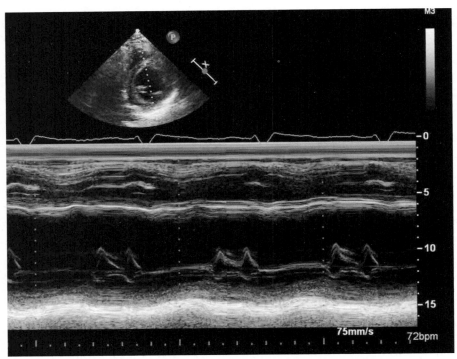

FIGURE 15-1. Increased mitral E point to septal separation in dilated cardiomyopathy.

- Two-dimensional and three-dimensional echo techniques are used to determine end-diastolic and end-systolic left ventricular volumes. This is then used to calculate left ventricular ejection fraction.
- Another useful measure of global systolic left ventricular function is dP/dt. It calculates the time that it takes the left ventricle to generate 32 mm Hg. The shorter the time, the better the function.
- Global longitudinal strain is increasingly being used as a quantitative measure of left ventricular function in cancer patients undergoing certain chemotherapy regimens.
- Ischemic versus nonischemic etiology:
  - It is useful to know whether a dilated cardiomyopathy is ischemic or nonischemic. Hence, an inquiry about prior cardiac catheterization is always warranted.
  - With an ischemic cardiomyopathy, the presence of certain regional left ventricular wall motion abnormalities may help decide when to repeat a coronary angiogram.
  - Patients with nonischemic cardiomyopathy may have regional wall motion abnormalities on echo without underlying coronary artery disease.
  - The preserved wall motion in nonischemic cardiomyopathy may be confined to the inferior and/or lateral walls.

- By knowing that the etiology is nonischemic, the existing wall motion abnormalities are not used improperly for decisions related to coronary artery disease.

Dennis AT, Castro JM. Echocardiographic differences between preeclampsia and peripartum cardiomyopathy. Int J Obstet Anesth. 2014;23:260–266.

An illustration of the key role of echocardiography in cardiomyopathies: Transthoracic echo enables differentiation of heart failure with preserved ejection fraction, commonly observed in women with preeclampsia, from that with peripartum cardiomyopathy, in which a reduced ejection fraction is more common.

- Sphericity:
  - The combination of decreased systolic ejection fraction with left ventricular dilatation creates a change in left ventricular geometry.
  - Over time, there is a disproportionate increase in the short axis, with a lesser increase in the long axis. This results in a progressive increase in sphericity. The left ventricle goes from "bullet to beach ball."
  - The echocardiographic consequence of the changed geometry is functional mitral regurgitation. Mitral leaflet coaptation becomes adversely affected by the reorientation of the papillary muscles in the left ventricle (due to the geometric changes).
- Scanning tip:
  - Caution when evaluating diastolic filling in dilated cardiomyopathy. Do not automatically use the left ventricular apex for reference.
  - In a dilated cardiomyopathy the cardiac apex may not be aligned with mitral inflow.
  - Pulsed-wave Doppler interrogation of mitral inflow at the leaflet tips should be parallel to the diastolic color flow jet. Therefore, the apical view needs to be adjusted and modified as needed.

Appleton CP, Jensen JL, Hatle LK, et al. Doppler evaluation of left and right ventricular diastolic function: a **technical guide** for obtaining optimal flow velocity recordings. Am Soc Echocardiogr. 1997;10:271–292.

DIASTOLIC ABNORMALITIES IN DILATED CARDIOMYOPATHY

- A restrictive left ventricular filling pattern (Fig. 15-2) in patients with dilated cardiomyopathy can be interpreted as follows:
  - The left atrial pressure is elevated.
  - The isovolumic relaxation time is shortened by the elevated left atrial pressure.
  - The mitral valve is being opened by the elevated left atrial pressures (not by mitral annular descent/suction).
  - Diastolic e' velocity is decreased due to abnormal diastolic function.
  - A normal e' velocity indicates *preserved* diastolic "suction."
  - Once e' is decreased in DCM, left atrial pressure rises and "pushes" blood into the left ventricle.

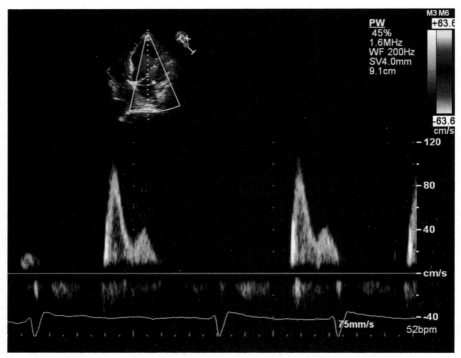

FIGURE 15-2. Restrictive left ventricular filling pattern. Pulsed-wave Doppler at the mitral leaflet tips.

- As a result:
  - The mitral inflow E velocity is increased.
  - Left atrial size progressively increases to act as a reservoir.
  - Caution: A restrictive left ventricular filling pattern should not be confused with a restrictive cardiomyopathy.

RESTRICTIVE CARDIOMYOPATHIES

Amyloid

"Heart in molasses"

- Echocardiographic findings in cardiac amyloidosis:
  - Subjectively sluggish systolic motion of the left ventricle (due to the myocardial infiltration).
  - Abnormal pulsed-wave tissue Doppler of the mitral annulus showing slow myocardial velocities.
  - Paradoxical low QRS voltage on the ECG, with evident left ventricular hypertrophy on echo.
  - Abnormally decreased basal and mid left ventricular longitudinal strain, with sparing of the left ventricular apex.
  - Abnormal longitudinal strain of the right ventricle.

*Bellavia D, Pellikka PA, Dispenzieri A, et al. Comparison of **right ventricular** longitudinal strain imaging, tricuspid annular plane systolic excursion, and cardiac biomarkers for early diagnosis of cardiac involvement and risk stratification in primary systematic (AL) amyloidosis: a 5-year cohort study. Eur Heart J Cardiovasc Imaging. 2012;13:680–689.*

*Buss SJ, Emami M, Mereles D, et al. Longitudinal left ventricular function for prediction of **survival** in systemic light-chain amyloidosis: incremental value compared with clinical and biochemical markers. J Am Coll Cardiol. 2012;60:1067–1076.*

*Koyama J, Ray-Sequin PA, Falk RH. Longitudinal myocardial function assessed by tissue velocity, **strain**, and strain rate tissue Doppler echocardiography in patients with AL (primary) cardiac amyloidosis. Circulation. 2003;107:2446–2452.*

*Phelan D, Collier P, Thavendiranathan P, et al. Relative **apical sparing** of longitudinal strain using two-dimensional speckle-tracking echocardiography is both sensitive and specific for the diagnosis of cardiac amyloidosis. Heart. 2012;98:1442–1448.*

IDIOPATHIC RESTRICTIVE CARDIOMYOPATHY

- This is a rare diagnosis of exclusion when other causes for cardiomyopathy have been excluded (no connective tissue disease, carcinoid syndrome, amyloidosis, hemochromatosis, eosinophilic syndrome, cancer, radiation therapy, cardiotoxic drug exposure, or alcohol abuse).
- There is mild to severe interstitial fibrosis, and mild myocyte hypertrophy on endomyocardial biopsy.
- This results in limited diastolic stretch capability, without left ventricular dilatation.
- Echo shows:
  - Small left ventricular diastolic chamber dimensions.
  - Preserved long-axis left ventricular function in two-thirds of patients.
  - Biatrial enlargement.
- A markedly dilated left atrium in an older female patient with this condition may indicate a poor prognosis.

*Perugini E, Rapezzi C, Reggiani LB, et al. **Comparison** of ventricular long-axis function in patients with cardiac amyloidosis versus idiopathic restrictive cardiomyopathy. Am J Cardiol. 2005;95:146–149.*

*Russo LM, Webber SA. Idiopathic restrictive cardiomyopathy in **children**. Heart. 2005;91:1199–1202.*

*Seward JB, Casaclang-Verzosa G. Infiltrative cardiovascular diseases: cardiomyopathies that **look alike**. J Am Coll Cardiol. 2010;55:1769–1779.*

ENDOMYOCARDIAL FIBROSIS

- Endomyocardial fibrosis is a *tropical zone* disease of unknown etiology.
- There is fibrous tissue on the endocardium and, to a lesser extent, in the myocardium of the inflow tract and apex of one or both ventricles.
- There is endocardial rigidity, atrioventricular valve incompetence secondary to papillary muscle involvement, and progressive reduction of the cavity of the involved ventricle leading to restriction in filling, and to atrial enlargement.
- A large portion of the apical left ventricle may be occupied by a thrombus.
- The "merlon" sign is a hypercontractile basal ventricle opposing an obliterated apex.
- Hepatic veins show a markedly deep diastolic forward wave throughout the respiratory cycle, and a marked reversal with inspiration.

Berensztein CS, Piñeiro D, Marcotegui M, et al. **Usefulness** *of echocardiography and Doppler echocardiography in endomyocardial fibrosis. J Am Soc Echocardiogr. 2000;13:385–392.*

Extensive description of the echocardiographic findings.

Hassan WM, Fawzy ME, Al Helaly S, et al. **Pitfalls** *in diagnosis and clinical, echocardiographic, and hemodynamic findings in endomyocardial fibrosis: a 25-year experience. Chest. 2005;128:3985–3992.*

Large left atrium. Small left ventricle. Obliteration of the apex.

FRIEDREICH ATAXIA

- Neuromuscular autosomal recessive disorder. Spinocerebellar degeneration.
- Patients develop a hypertrophic or, less commonly, a dilated cardiomyopathy.

Alboliras ET, Shub C, Gomez MR, et al. Spectrum of cardiac involvement in Friedreich's ataxia: clinical, electrocardiographic and **echocardiographic** *observations. Am J Cardiol. 1986;58:518–524.*

Hanson E, Sheldon M, Pacheco B, et al. **Heart disease** *in Friedreich's ataxia. World J Cardiol. 2019;11:1–12.*

Weidemann F, Störk S, Liu D, et al. **Cardiomyopathy** *of Friedreich ataxia. J Neurochem. 2013;126 Suppl 1:88–93.*

RADIATION-INDUCED HEART DISEASE

- Patients can develop transient pericardial effusions a few weeks after radiation.
- The pericardial effusion may recur 6 to 12 months after radiation.
- Constrictive pericarditis may develop.
- There may be valvular fibrosis with color flow evidence of valvular regurgitation.
- A restrictive cardiomyopathy may develop with:
  - Decreased left ventricular size.
  - Reduced wall thickness.
  - Decreased left ventricular systolic function.
  - Diastolic dysfunction.
  - Fibrosis of the right ventricular free wall.
- Radiation-induced heart disease is most commonly found in Hodgkin disease survivors.
- Other cancer survivors with this complication have been treated for non-Hodgkin lymphomas, esophageal carcinoma, thymoma, lung cancer, breast cancer, and metastatic seminoma.
- Risk factors:
  - Previous chemotherapy.
  - Radiation exposure exceeding 4000 rad.
  - Radiation close to the heart, and on the left side of the chest.
- Patients may develop disease of the proximal coronary arteries, especially if they have risk factors for coronary artery disease.

Brosius FC, Waller BF, Roberts WC. Radiation heart disease. Analysis of 16 young (aged 15 to 33 years) necropsy patients who received over 3,500 rads to the heart. Am J Med. 1981;70:519–530.

Carlson RG, Mayfield WR, Normann S, et al. Radiation-associated **valvular** disease. Chest. 1991;99:538–545.

Cheng RK, Lee MS, Seki A, et al. Radiation **coronary arteritis** refractory to surgical and percutaneous revascularization culminating in orthotopic heart transplantation. Cardiovasc Pathol. 2013;22:303–308.

Darby SC, Cutter DJ, Boerma M, et al. Radiation-related heart disease: current knowledge and **future** prospects. Int J Radiat Oncol Biol Phys. 2010;76:656–665.

Filopei J, Frishman W. Radiation-induced heart disease. Cardiol Rev. 2012;20:184–188.

Glanzmann C, Kaufmann P, Jenni R, et al. Cardiac risk after mediastinal irradiation for Hodgkin's disease. Radiother Oncol. 1998;46:51–62.

Gustavsson A, Eskilsson T, Landberg T, et al. Late cardiac effects after mantle radiotherapy in patients with **Hodgkin's** disease. Ann Oncol. 1990;1:355–363.

Han X, Zhou Y, Liu W. Precision cardio-oncology: understanding the cardiotoxicity of cancer therapy. NPJ Precis Oncol. 2017;1:31.

Heidenreich PA, Hancock SL, Lee BK, et al. **Asymptomatic** cardiac disease following mediastinal irradiation. J Am Coll Cardiol. 2003;42:743–749.

Screening echocardiography should be considered for patients with a history of mediastinal irradiation.

Heidenreich PA, Hancock SL, Vagelos RH, et al. **Diastolic** dysfunction after mediastinal irradiation. Am Heart J. 2005;150:977–982.

There is a high prevalence of diastolic dysfunction in asymptomatic patients after mediastinal irradiation.

King V, Constine LS, Clark D, et al. Symptomatic coronary artery disease after mantle irradiation for Hodgkin's disease. Int J Radiat Oncol Biol Phys. 1996;36:881–889.

Lipshultz SE, Lipsitz SR, Sallan SE, et al. Chronic progressive cardiac dysfunction years after **doxorubicin** therapy for childhood acute lymphoblastic leukemia. J Clin Oncol. 2005;23:2629–2636.

McGale P, Darby SC, Hall P, et al. Incidence of heart disease in 35,000 women treated with radiotherapy for **breast cancer** in Denmark and Sweden. Radiother Oncol. 2011;100:167–175.

Piovaccari G, Ferretti RM, Prati F, et al. Cardiac disease after chest irradiation for **Hodgkin's** disease: incidence in 108 patients with long follow-up. Int J Cardiol. 1995;49:39–43.

Veinot JP, Edwards WD. Pathology of radiation-induced heart disease: a surgical and autopsy study of 27 cases. Hum Pathol. 1996;27:766–773.

NONCOMPACTION

"Excessively prominent trabecular meshwork and deep intertrabecular recesses because of an arrest of compaction of the meshwork of myocardial fibers during intrauterine life."

- In normal cardiac development:
  - The myocardium condenses and the intertrabecular recesses are reduced to capillaries.
  - The ratio of noncompacted to compacted myocardium is measured in the short-axis views with contrast enhancement.

de Groot-de Laat LE, Krenning BJ, ten Cate FJ, et al. Usefulness of **contrast** *echocardiography for diagnosis of left ventricular noncompaction. Am J Cardiol. 2005;95:1131–1134.*

Jenni R, Oechslin E, Schneider J, et al. Echocardiographic and pathoanatomical **characteristics** *of isolated left ventricular non-compaction: a step towards classification as a distinct cardiomyopathy. Heart. 2001;86:666–671.*

Song ZZ. Echocardiography in the **diagnosis** *left ventricular noncompaction. Cardiovasc Ultrasound. 2008;6:64.*

SARCOIDOSIS

"An inflammatory multisystem disease."

- Cardiac involvement should be suspected in *advanced* cases.
- Echo looks for pericardial and myocardial involvement.
- Diastolic dysfunction may be present.
- Restrictive cardiomyopathy is *uncommon* in sarcoidosis.
- Mitral regurgitation is common but nonspecific.
- Left ventricular wall motion abnormalities may not follow a coronary artery distribution.
- Ventricular septal thickness may be increased during *early stages*—possibly due to myocardial cell infiltration or edema.
- Cardiac sarcoidosis may be misdiagnosed as arrhythmogenic right ventricular dysplasia.

Fahy GJ, Marwick T, McCreery CJ, et al. Doppler echocardiographic detection of left ventricular **diastolic** *dysfunction in patients with pulmonary sarcoidosis. Chest. 1996;109:62–66.*

Diastolic dysfunction was present in 7 (14%) patients, 6 of whom had normal systolic function and normal two-dimensional echocardiographic examination. Those with diastolic dysfunction had a longer duration of illness, were significantly older, and had higher systolic BP than the sarcoid patients with normal diastolic function.

Okamura H, Goto Y, Terashima M, et al. Reversible **right ventricular** *hypertrophy due to cardiac sarcoidosis. Circulation. 2005;111:e383–e384.*

Slart RHJA, Glaudemans AWJM, Lancellotti P, et al. A joint procedural position statement on **imaging** *in cardiac sarcoidosis. J Nucl Cardiol. 2018;25:298–319.*

ARRHYTHMOGENIC RIGHT VENTRICULAR CARDIOMYOPATHY

- Arrhythmogenic right ventricular cardiomyopathy (dysplasia) is a predominantly right ventricular disorder.
- Pathology shows replacement of myocardial fibers with fatty, fibrous, or fibrofatty tissue.
- Echocardiographic findings:
  - Sacculations of the right ventricular free wall.
  - Dilatation of the right ventricle, and right ventricular outflow.
  - Myocardial thinning and dyskinesis.
  - Thickening and hyperreflectivity of the moderator band.

Deshpande SR, Herman HK, Quigley PC, et al. Arrhythmogenic right ventricular cardiomyopathy/dysplasia (ARVC/D): review of 16 pediatric cases and a proposal of modified **pediatric** criteria. Pediatr Cardiol. 2016;37:646–655.

Marcus FI, McKenna WJ, Sherrill D, et al. **Diagnosis** of arrhythmogenic right ventricular cardiomyopathy/dysplasia: proposed modification of the task force criteria. Circulation. 2010;121:1533–1541.

Pinamonti B, Pagnan L, Bussani R, et al. Right ventricular dysplasia with biventricular involvement. Circulation. 1998;98: 1943–1945.

Yoerger DM, Marcus F, Sherrill D, et al. Echocardiographic **findings** in patients meeting task force criteria for arrhythmogenic right ventricular dysplasia: new insights from the multidisciplinary study of right ventricular dysplasia. J Am Coll Cardiol. 2005;45:860–865.

APICAL BALLOONING SYNDROME

Lyon AR, Bossone E, Schneider B, et al. Current **state of knowledge** on Takotsubo syndrome. Eur J Heart Fail. 2016; 18:8–27.

- Echocardiographic findings:
- Acute phase:
  - Large area of dysfunctional myocardium.
  - Extension beyond the territory of a single coronary artery.
  - Symmetrical regional abnormalities involving the mid ventricular segments of the anterior, inferior, and lateral walls (a circumferential pattern).
- Complications:
  - LV outflow obstruction.
  - LV thrombus.
  - Mitral regurgitation.
  - Right ventricular involvement.
  - Cardiac rupture.
- Major adverse events (acute heart failure, cardiogenic shock, and in hospital death) predicted by:
  - Low LVEF.
  - Elevated E/e' ratio.
  - Reversible moderate to severe mitral regurgitation.
  - Age ≥75 years.
- Contrast may be useful in understanding microvascular function in this disorder.

Abdelmoneim SS, Mankad SV, Bernier M, et al. **Microvascular** function in Takotsubo cardiomyopathy with contrast echocardiography: prospective evaluation and review of literature. J Am Soc Echo. 2009;22:1249–1255.

CHAGAS MYOCARDITIS

- Chagas disease is due to infection by *Trypanosoma cruzi*.
- Classic echo finding: large narrow-neck apical left ventricular aneurysm.
- Most common echo finding: global left ventricular dysfunction.
- History of travel to endemic regions in South America is key to suspecting the diagnosis.

GUIDELINES

Acquatella H, Asch FM, Barbosa MM, et al. Recommendations for multimodality cardiac imaging in patients with Chagas disease. J Am Soc Echocardiogr. 2018;31:3–25.

Nunes MCP, Badano LP, Marin-Neto JA, et al. Multimodality imaging evaluation of Chagas disease. Eur Heart J Cardiovasc Imaging. 2018;19:459–460.

- These two guideline documents complement each other.
- Numerous scanning pointers are provided.
- Cardiac imaging is crucial for the care of these patients.
- Strain is useful.
- There are examples of typical apical aneurysms.
- Echo is useful during all stages of the disease.

RHEUMATOID ARTHRITIS

- Global longitudinal LV and RV strain is reduced in patients with RA compared with healthy patients.
- Strain abnormalities correlate with RA disease severity.
- Strain imaging by echocardiography may detect early myocardial dysfunction in RA.

Fine NM, Crowson CS, Lin G, et al. Evaluation of myocardial function in patients with rheumatoid arthritis using strain imaging by speckle-tracking echocardiography. Ann Rheum Dis. 2014;73:1833–1839.

PERICARDIAL CONSTRICTION

- Constricting pericardium creates a *shell* around the heart.
- Intracardiac and intrathoracic pressure changes become dissociated. This provides the hemodynamic foundation for the echocardiographic diagnosis of constriction.
- The fixed constricted cardiac volume cannot adapt. When one ventricle fills, the other one pays a price.
- On inspiration, the diaphragm creates an intrathoracic vacuum with a pressure drop.
- Intrathoracic pressure changes are not transmitted to the cardiac chambers evenly because of the constricting pericardial shell.
- In constriction, on inspiration, intrathoracic pulmonary vein pressure drops, but intracardiac left atrial pressure does not. As a result, there is less forward flow from the pulmonary veins to the left atrium—left heart filling decreases on inspiration in constriction.
- Echocardiographic translation:
  - Mitral inflow decreases on inspiration.
  - In constriction, there is a drop in mitral E velocity on inspiration, along with a brief early diastolic restrictive filling pattern.
  - There is a respiratory bounce of the interventricular septum, as the left ventricle "pays the price" for increased inspiratory right ventricular filling.
  - This is corrected on expiration, manifested as expiratory flow reversal in the hepatic veins (Figs. 16-9 and 16-10).

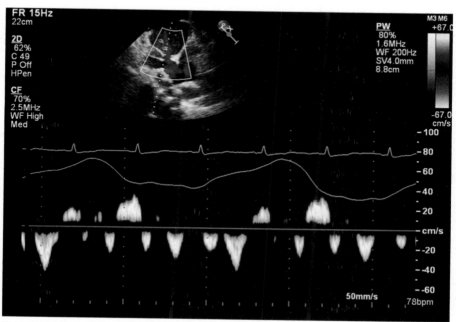

FIGURE 16-9. Expiratory reversal of hepatic vein flow in pericardial constriction.

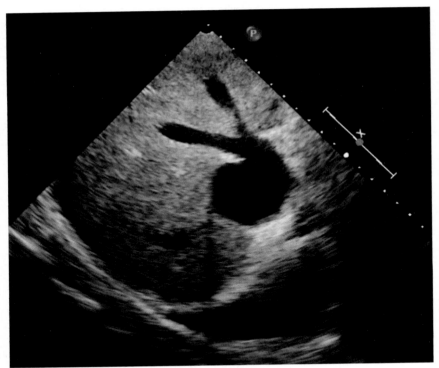

FIGURE 16-10. Dilated hepatic vein. Bunny sign.

- The tissue Doppler e' velocity helps distinguish the heart failure of constriction from other forms of heart failure where myocardium, rather than pericardium, is responsible for heart failure.

*Ginghina C, Beladan CC, Iancu M, et al. **Respiratory maneuvers** in echocardiography: a review of clinical applications. Cardiovasc Ultrasound. 2009;7:42.*

Ha JW, Oh JK, Ling LH, et al. Annulus paradoxus: transmitral flow velocity to mitral annular velocity ratio is inversely proportional to pulmonary capillary wedge pressure in patients with constrictive pericarditis. Circulation. 2001;104:976–978.

The lateral expansion of the heart is limited by constricting pericardium, resulting in exaggerated longitudinal motion of the mitral annulus. The more severe the constriction, the more accentuated the longitudinal motion.

*Jottrand E, Serste T, Mulkay JP, et al. Longitudinal **strain** by speckle tracking echocardiography in constrictive pericarditis. Eur Heart J Cardiovasc Imaging. 2018;19:638.*

The typical strain deformation pattern of the left ventricle in constrictive pericarditis includes:

- *Preserved longitudinal **septal** strain.*
- *Reduced longitudinal left ventricular **free wall** strain due to pericardial adhesions.*

Ling LH, Oh JK, Tei C, et al. Pericardial thickness measured with transesophageal echocardiography: feasibility and potential clinical usefulness. J Am Coll Cardiol. 1997;29:1317.

Oh JK, Tajik AJ, Appleton CP, et al. Preload reduction to unmask the characteristic Doppler features of constrictive pericarditis. A new observation. Circulation. 1997;95:796–799.

When the respiratory variation in Doppler mitral E velocity is blunted or absent during the evaluation of suspected constrictive pericarditis, repeat Doppler recording of mitral flow velocities after maneuvers to decrease preload is recommended to unmask the characteristic respiratory variation in mitral E velocity.

Sengupta PP, Mohan JC, Mehta V, et al. Accuracy and pitfalls of early diastolic motion of the mitral annulus for diagnosing constrictive pericarditis by tissue Doppler imaging. Am J Cardiol. 2004;93:886–890.

Mitral annular velocities help with diagnosis and differentiation of constrictive pericarditis in most cases, except in the presence of extensive annular calcification, left ventricular systolic dysfunction, or segmental nonuniformity in myocardial velocities.

EPICARDIAL FAT

- Pericardial fat may manifest as an echolucent "stripe" that does not change in size with body position (does not "layer out" with gravity).
- In morbidly obese patients, there are multiple parallel stripes anterior to the right ventricular outflow in the PLAX view.
- There are no matching stripes posterior to the heart in these patients, but an unrelated pericardial effusion may be present.

Haaz WS, Mintz GS, Kotler MN, et al. 2-Dimensional echocardiographic recognition of the descending thoracic aorta—value in differentiating pericardial from pleural effusions. Am J Cardiol. 1980;46:739–743 (Figs. 16-11 and 16-12).

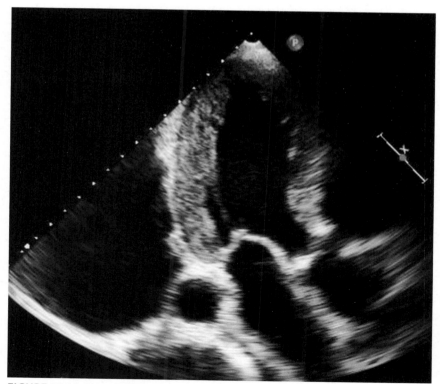

FIGURE 16-11. Pleural effusion that extends behind the aorta.

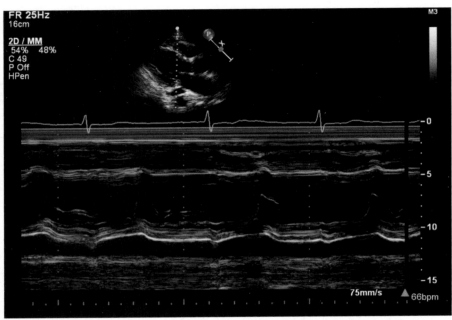

FIGURE 16-12. A dilated coronary sinus should not be mistaken for a pericardial effusion on M-mode.

The location of the descending thoracic aorta on two-dimensional echocardiography serves as a landmark in localizing the pericardial–pleural interface, thereby helping to differentiate pericardial from pleural effusions.

- Epicardial fat is commonly visualized in PLAX and SAX.
- Echocardiographic epicardial fat thickness ranges from 1 mm to as much as 23 mm, and may sometimes be difficult to differentiate from pericardial fluid.
- It appears as an echo-free space between the outer wall of the myocardium and the visceral layer of the pericardium.
- Epicardial fat appears to move *in tandem* with the adjacent myocardium.
- It is measured perpendicularly on the outside of the free wall of the right ventricle at end-systole.
- It reflects visceral adiposity rather than general obesity and may correlate with metabolic syndrome, insulin resistance, coronary artery disease, and subclinical atherosclerosis.

*Iacobellis G, Willens HJ. Echocardiographic **epicardial fat**: a review of research and clinical applications. J Am Soc Echocardiogr. 2009;22:1311–1319.*

INTERVENTIONAL PROCEDURES FOR PERICARDIAL DISEASES

- Drainage of pericardial effusion.
- Intrapericardial therapy/sclerosis of the pericardial space.

- Percutaneous balloon pericardiotomy.
- Pericardiocentesis.
- Devices for pericardiocentesis: PerDUCER, PeriAttacher, visual puncture systems, grasper, scissors, reverse slitter.

Maisch B, Ristić AD, Pankuweit S, et al. Percutaneous therapy in pericardial diseases. Cardiol Clin. 2017;35:567–588.

EFFUSIVE CONSTRICTIVE PERICARDITIS

- Uncommon pericardial syndrome that may be missed in some tamponade patients.
- There is a tense pericardial effusion, but there is also concomitant constriction by the pericardium. Simply put, the pericardium behaves like a SCUBA diving wetsuit.
- After pericardiocentesis, the intrapericardial pressure decreases, but right atrial and end-diastolic right and left ventricular pressures remain elevated.
- The visceral layer of the pericardium needs to be removed surgically.

Hancock EW. Subacute effusive-constrictive pericarditis. Circulation. 1971;43:183–192.

Sagrista-Sauleda J, Angel J, Sanchez A, et al. Effusive-constrictive pericarditis. N Engl J Med. 2004;350:469–475.

Sagrista-Sauleda J, Permanyer-Miralda G, Candell-Riera J, et al. Transient cardiac constriction—an unrecognized pattern of evolution in effusive acute idiopathic pericarditis. Am J Cardiol. 1987;59:961–966.

PERICARDIECTOMY

- Once the diagnosis of constrictive pericarditis (CP) is made, the patient may be referred for pericardiectomy.
- The surgery can alleviate or improve heart failure symptoms.
- Long-term survival after pericardiectomy for CP is related to underlying etiology.
- There is relatively good survival with idiopathic constrictive pericarditis.
- Long-term results of pericardiectomy may be disappointing with radiation-induced constrictive pericarditis.
- Preoperative heart failure is associated with lower long-term survival.
- Caution: The chest pain of pericarditis may not resolve after pericardiectomy in some patients.

Bertog SC, Thambidorai SK, Parakh K, et al. Constrictive pericarditis: etiology and cause-specific survival after **pericardiectomy**. J Am Coll Cardiol. 2004;43:1445–1452.

Dhar SC, Hayes S, Cercek B, et al. Images in cardiovascular medicine. Cardiac **tuberculosis**. Circulation. 1998;98:730.

George TJ, Arnaoutakis GJ, Beaty CA, et al. Contemporary etiologies, risk factors, and outcomes after **pericardiectomy**. Ann Thorac Surg. 2012;94:445–451.

Ling LH, Oh JK, Schaff HV, et al. Constrictive pericarditis in the modern era: evolving clinical spectrum and impact on outcome after **pericardiectomy**. Circulation. 1999;100:1380–1386.

Mutyaba AK, Balkaran S, Cloete R, et al. Constrictive pericarditis requiring **pericardiectomy** at Groote Schuur Hospital, Cape Town, South Africa: causes and perioperative outcomes in the HIV era (1990–2012). J Thorac Cardiovasc Surg. 2014;148: 3058–3065.

Szabo G, Schmack B, Bulut C, et al. Constrictive pericarditis: risks, aetiologies and outcomes after total **pericardiectomy**: 24 years of experience. Eur J Cardiothorac Surg. 2013;44:1023–1028.

PULMONARY REGURGITATION IN CONSTRICTION

- The Doppler signal of pulmonic valve regurgitation depends on the relationship between pulmonary artery (intrathoracic) and right ventricular (intracardiac) pressure.
- Early diastolic cessation with inspiration correctly diagnosed constrictive pericarditis in 70% of patients in the study below.

Gilman G, Ommen SR, Hansen WH, et al. Doppler echocardiographic evaluation of pulmonary regurgitation facilitates the diagnosis of constrictive pericarditis. J Am Soc Echocardiogr. 2005;18:892–895.

DRESSLER SYNDROME

- This is a pericardial effusion syndrome that follows cardiac injury.
- Manifestations:
  - Pericardial effusion.
  - Fever.
  - Clinical evidence of pericarditis (chest pain, rub on auscultation, typical pericarditis ECG).
  - Sequel to myocardial infarction, cardiac surgery, chest trauma, pacemaker insertion.
  - Latency time of weeks to months.
- Other manifestations:
  - Pleural effusion.
  - Tamponade.
  - Evolution to pericardial constriction.

Beaufils P, Bardet J, Temkine J, et al. Dressler's syndrome: constrictive pericarditis following myocardial infarction operated on with success. Arch Mal Coeur Vaiss. 1975;68:651–656.

Cevik C, Wilborn T, Corona R, et al. Post-cardiac injury syndrome following transvenous pacemaker insertion: a case report and review of the literature. Heart Lung Circ. 2009;18:379–383.

Dressler W. A post-myocardial infarction syndrome; preliminary report of a complication resembling idiopathic, recurrent, benign pericarditis. JAMA. 1956;160:1379–1383.

Dressler W. The post-myocardial-infarction syndrome: a report on forty-four cases. AMA Arch Intern Med. 1959;103:28–42.

Hertzeanu H, Almog C, Algom M. Cardiac tamponade in Dressler's syndrome. Case report. Cardiology. 1983;70:31–36.

Imazio M, Hoit BD. Post-cardiac injury syndromes. An emerging cause of pericardial diseases. Int J Cardiol. 2013;168:648.

Paelinck B, Dendale PA. Images in clinical medicine. Cardiac tamponade in Dressler's syndrome. N Engl J Med. 2003;348:e8.

Wessman DE, Stafford CM. The postcardiac injury syndrome: case report and review of the literature. South Med J. 2006;99:309–314.

Nine cases were reported following pacemaker implantation between 1975 and 2009. Symptoms appeared 5–56 days after the procedure. All had pleuropericardial involvement. Six cases improved with medical therapy. Three required a pericardial window.

PERICARDIAL CYST

- A developmental abnormality.
- Round or oval appearance.
- Thin walled.
- Loculated.
- Filled with clear fluid.
- Most common location: right cardiophrenic angle, adjacent to the cardiac border.
- Utility of echocardiography:
    - Confirm the echo-free content of the cyst.
    - Doppler flow and saline contrast are used to confirm no blood flow in the cyst.
    - Serial echo imaging is used for follow-up.
    - Echo can guide needle aspiration if there is a compressive effect by the cyst.
    - Note: Pericardial cyst fluid tends to reaccumulate after needle aspiration.
    - Thoracoscopic surgical removal is usually needed for definitive treatment.
- Differential diagnosis:
    - Pericardial diverticulum.
    - Loculated pericardial effusion.
    - Diaphragmatic hernia.

Kar SK, Ganguly T. Current concepts of diagnosis and management of pericardial cysts. Indian Heart J. 2017;69:364–370.

Money ME, Park C. Pericardial diverticula misdiagnosed as pericardial cysts. J Thorac Cardiovasc Surg. 2015;149:e103–e107.

*Pericardial cysts result from complete closure of an embryonic pericardial defect. However, 10% of all cysts may instead be a **pericardial diverticulum** with a persistent connection to the pericardial space.*

Najib MQ, Chaliki HP, Raizada A, et al. Symptomatic pericardial cyst: a case series. Eur J Echocardiogr. 2011;12:E43.

Patel J, Park C, Michaels J, et al. Pericardial cyst: case reports and a literature review. Echocardiography. 2004 21:269–272.

CONGENITAL PARTIAL OR COMPLETE ABSENCE OF THE PERICARDIUM

- Cardiac magnetic resonance imaging is currently the standard for diagnosis.
- Echocardiographic findings that should suggest the diagnosis:
    - Unusual echocardiographic windows.
    - Cardiac hypermobility.
    - Abnormal ventricular septal motion.
    - Abnormal swinging motion of the heart.
    - Teardrop left ventricle.
    - Elongated atria.

- In rare cases, herniation and strangulation of cardiac chambers can be life threatening and can lead to sudden cardiac death.

Abbas AE, Appleton CP, Liu PT, et al. *Congenital absence of the pericardium: case presentation and review of literature.* Int J Cardiol. 2005;98:21–25.

Connolly HM, Click RL, Schattenberg TT, et al. *Congenital absence of the pericardium: echocardiography as a diagnostic tool.* J Am Soc Echocardiogr. 1995;8:87–92.

Foo JS, Koh CH, Sahlén A, et al. *Congenital partial absence of pericardium: a mimic of arrhythmogenic right ventricular cardiomyopathy.* Case Rep Med. 2018;2018:4297280.

Shah AB, Kronzon I. *Congenital defects of the pericardium: a review.* Eur Heart J Cardiovasc Imaging. 2015;16:821–827.

VIDEOS

VIDEO 16-1 (A–E). Right ventricular free wall diastolic compression and partial inversion.

VIDEO 16-2. M-mode of right ventricular free wall inversion.

VIDEO 16-3 (A–H). Right atrial inversion.

VIDEO 16-4. Pericardial effusion after pacemaker insertion. Elevated right atrial pressure due to pacemaker wire–induced tricuspid regurgitation, may explain absence of right atrial inversion.

VIDEO 16-5. Right atrial and right ventricular inversion.

VIDEO 16-6. Left atrial inversion.

VIDEO 16-7. Biatrial inversion in tamponade.

VIDEO 16-8 (A–E). Respiratory bounce of the interventricular septum. Pericardial constriction.

VIDEO 16-9 (A,B). Fluoroscopic appearance of calcified pericardium.

VIDEO 16-10 (A,B). Cardiac translation ("swinging heart"). There may be electrical QRS alternans on the ECG.

VIDEO 16-11. Large pericardial effusion.

VIDEO 16-12. Large pericardial effusion. The right ventricle appears to turn in systole.

VIDEO 16-13. Large predominantly posterior pericardial effusion.

VIDEO 16-14. Moderate pericardial effusion.

VIDEO 16-15 (A,B). Small pericardial effusion.

VIDEO 16-16. Multiple views may be needed to distinguish pleural and pericardial effusions.

VIDEO 16-17 (A,B). Small pericardial effusion and a pleural effusion. Descending aorta serves as a landmark.

VIDEO 16-18. Pericardial (not pleural) effusion interposed between the coronary sinus and the descending aorta.

VIDEO 16-19. Pericardial fluid in the transverse sinus, between the posterior wall of the aorta and the left atrial wall.

VIDEO 16-20 (A–C). Typical triangular shape of pericardial fluid in the transverse sinus on TEE.

VIDEO 16-21. Fibrin in the transverse sinus.

VIDEO 16-22 (A–C). Reverberation artifact caused by epicardial fibrin.

VIDEO 16-23. Pericardial reverberation artifact.

VIDEO 16-24. Pericardial thickness illustrated by surrounding pleural fluid and intrapericardial fluid.

VIDEO 16-25. Mildly increased pericardial thickness.

VIDEO 16-26. The pericardium is the brightest reflection in this image.

VIDEO 16-27 (A–C). Intrapericardial fibrin.

VIDEO 16-28 (A,B). Fibrinous pericardial effusion.

VIDEO 16-29. Fibrinous pericardial fluid (not epicardial fat) anterior to the right ventricle.

VIDEO 16-30 (A–D). Intrapericardial thrombus following open heart surgery.

VIDEO 16-31. Intrapericardial thrombus and respiratory "bounce" of the interventricular septum.

VIDEO 16-32. Right atrial compression by an intrapericardial thrombus following open heart surgery.

VIDEO 16-33. Interposed hepatic parenchyma precludes needle aspiration of pericardial effusion.

VIDEO 16-34 (A–D). Homogeneous nonfibrotic myocardium with no ultrasound reflections may be mistaken for pericardial fluid.

VIDEO 16-35. Contrast injected into the pericardial space.

VIDEO 16-36. Normal hepatic vein flow.

VIDEO 16-37. Normal hepatic vein flow with respiratory variation.

VIDEO 16-38. Inspiratory increase in hepatic vein flow.

VIDEO 16-39. Less than 50% decrease in IVC diameter with a sniff. No evident change in hepatic vein flow direction.

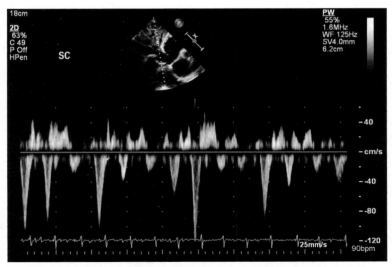

FIGURE 16-13. Abnormal but nondiagnostic hepatic vein flow. Increased diastolic velocities toward the heart. Intermittent systolic flow reversal.

VIDEO 16-40 (A,B). Hepatic vein flow. Color M-mode can be used for timing the reversals.

VIDEO 16-41. Normal brief late diastolic hepatic vein flow reversal after the atrial contraction. This is the Doppler equivalent of the jugular "a" wave on physical examination.

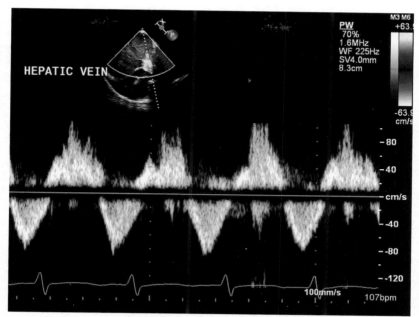

FIGURE 16-14. Hepatic vein systolic flow reversal in severe tricuspid regurgitation.

VIDEO 16-42. Hepatic vein systolic flow reversal in severe tricuspid regurgitation.

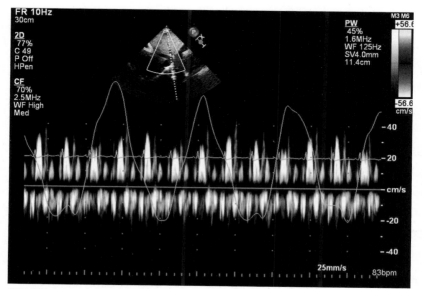

FIGURE 16-15. Expiratory hepatic vein flow reversal in pericardial constriction.

VIDEO 16-43. Diastolic dominant caval inflow.

VIDEO 16-44. Respiratory variation in caval inflow.

VIDEO 16-45. Normal respiratory variation in IVC diameter. Normal right atrial pressure.

VIDEO 16-46. No change in IVC diameter with a sniff. Elevated right atrial pressure.

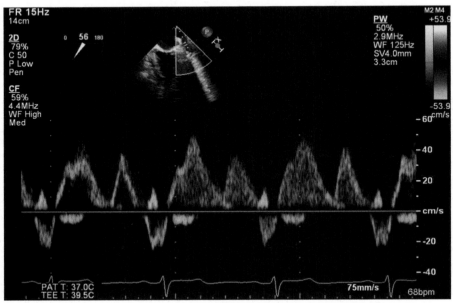

FIGURE 16-16. S1 and S2 pulmonary vein inflow waves. S1 is due to atrial relaxation. S2 is due to mitral annular descent.

VIDEO 16-47. Mirror artifact. Minimal pericardial effusion.

VIDEO 16-48. Minimal pericardial effusion.

VIDEO 16-49 (A–C). Pleural effusion.

VIDEO 16-50. Cardiac amyloidosis. The usual small pericardial effusion is absent. Instead, there is a pleural effusion that extends behind the descending aorta.

VIDEO 16-51. Pleural fibrin external to the pericardium.

VIDEO 16-52. Pleural fibrin.

VIDEO 16-53 (A–C). Increased distance between the transducer and the pericardium in morbidly obese patients.

VIDEO 16-54 (A,B). Normal pericardial thickness.

VIDEO 16-55. Normal pericardial thickness anterior to the right ventricle.

VIDEO 16-56. Arc-like artifact that can be mistaken for a pacemaker wire.

CHAPTER 17

Endocarditis

2015 GUIDELINES

Baddour LM, Wilson WR, Bayer AS, et al. Infective Endocarditis in Adults: Diagnosis, Antimicrobial Therapy, and Management of Complications: A Scientific Statement for Healthcare Professionals From the American Heart Association. Circulation. 2015;132:1435–1486.

- Echo is central to diagnosis and management.
- Echo findings may suggest a need for surgical intervention.
- Recommendations are made for initial and repeat echo imaging.

European Guidelines

Habib G, Hoen B, Tornos P, et al. Guidelines on the prevention, diagnosis, and treatment of infective endocarditis: The Task Force on the Prevention, Diagnosis, and Treatment of Infective Endocarditis of the European Society of Cardiology (ESC). Eur Heart J. 2009;30:2369–2413.

- Extensive document covering all clinical aspects of endocarditis.

DISEASE OVERVIEW

- Endocarditis is caused by, and accompanied by, bacteremia or fungemia.
- The echocardiographic hallmark is a vegetation.
- Microorganisms attract blood fibrin and platelets to form the vegetation.

Cahill TJ, Baddour LM, Habib G, et al. Challenges in Infective Endocarditis. J Am Coll Cardiol. 2017;69:325–344.

- Location of vegetations:
  - Most commonly attached to the surface of native valve leaflets.
  - May attach to mitral or tricuspid chordae.
  - Difficult to localize and diagnose on prosthetic valves.
- Pacemaker/ICD wires may have to be completely removed if they become infected.
- Congenital heart defects and congenital defect repairs may become infected.

- The point of *attachment* varies, but there are some useful typical echo features.
- Vegetations are said to favor the upstream side of valves: Atrial side of mitral and tricuspid valves, and ventricular side of aortic valves (pulmonic valve endocarditis is rare).
- The usual *appearance* is a shimmering, shaggy, stippled, pedunculated mass.
- Reflectivity and texture are typically similar to normal myocardium.
- Calcification suggests chronicity.

*Kini V, Logani S, Ky B, et al. Transthoracic and transesophageal echocardiography for the indication of suspected endocarditis: vegetations, blood cultures, and **imaging**. J Am Soc Echocardiogr. 2010;23:396–402.*

- Complications:
  - Leaflet perforation.
  - Abscess.
  - Fistula.
  - Embolism.

*Anguera I, Miro JM, Vilacosta I, et al. Aorto-cavitary **fistulous tract** formation in infective endocarditis: clinical and echocardiographic features of 76 cases and risk factors for mortality. Eur Heart J. 2005;26:288–297.*

*Sudhakar S, Sewani A, Agrawal M, et al. Pseudoaneurysm of the mitral-aortic **intervalvular fibrosa** (MAIVF): a comprehensive review. J Am Soc Echocardiogr. 2010;23:1009–1018.*

*Thuny F, Disalvo G, Belliard O, et al. Risk of **embolism** and death in infective endocarditis: prognostic value of echocardiography. A prospective multicenter study. Circulation. 2005;112:69–75.*

- Clinical suspicion:
  - Persistent fever.
  - Fever with a new murmur.
  - Change in an existing murmur.
  - Conduction abnormality on ECG.
  - Embolic event.
  - Newly diagnosed dehiscence on echo of an existing prosthetic valve.
  - New heart failure is an ominous finding and justifies surgical intervention.
- Differential diagnosis:
  - Calcification.
  - Lambl excrescences.
  - Libman-Sacks.
  - Blood cyst.
  - Ruptured chordae/flail leaflets.
- Vegetation size is related to prognosis.
- Fungal vegetations and tricuspid valve vegetations tend to be bigger (Fig. 17-1).
- Transesophageal echocardiography should be performed when high clinical suspicion remains after a negative or nondiagnostic transthoracic study.
- Echo is used to guide *duration* of antibiotic therapy.
- Indications for surgery:
  - New onset of heart failure.
  - Embolic event/stroke.

- Extension of infection/abscess.
- Endocarditis caused by fungi or other resistant organisms.
- Abscess.
- Increase in vegetation size.
- Clinically worse valvular regurgitation.
- Cardiac chamber enlargement.
- Worsening left ventricular dysfunction.
- New elevation in left ventricular filling pressure.
- Diagnostic criteria—patients are classified as:
  - Definite evidence of endocarditis.
  - Possible endocarditis.
  - Diagnosis rejected.

Durack DT, Lukes AS, Bright DK. **New criteria** for diagnosis of infective endocarditis: utilization of specific echocardiographic findings. Am J Med. 1994;96:200–209.

The Duke criteria incorporated echo in 1994.

Li JS, Sexton DJ, Mick N, et al. Proposed **modifications** to the Duke criteria for the diagnosis of infective endocarditis. Clin Infect Dis. 2000;30:633–638.

von Reyn CF, Levy BS, Arbeit RD, et al. Infective endocarditis: an analysis based on strict case definitions. Ann Intern Med. 1981;94:505–518.

von Reyn criteria for endocarditis. There were no echo criteria in 1981.

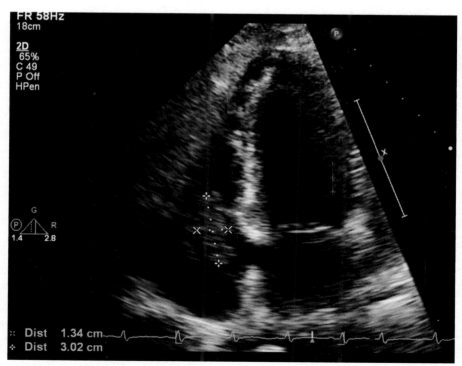

FIGURE 17-1. Tricuspid valve vegetation.

VALVULAR DESTRUCTION

- Severe *regurgitation* of infected aortic or mitral valves can cause heart failure, which is an indication for surgery in patients with endocarditis.
- Valve *perforation* occurs in infected bicuspid aortic valves because they are prone to abscess formation.
- An infected *saccular aneurysm* on the atrial aspect of the anterior mitral valve leaflet can perforate and create a windsock defect in the leaflet body.
- Scanning tip: Zoom in with 2D and 3D to look for a PISA entraining into the body of a perforated leaflet.
- Acute severe *aortic* valve regurgitation may show *diastolic mitral* valve regurgitation, mitral valve preclosure, and diastolic flow reversal in the descending thoracic aorta.
- Acute severe *mitral* valve regurgitation may show a restrictive left ventricular filling pattern, mitral regurgitation peak velocities below the usual 5 m/s, and truncation of the parabolic CW signal to a triangular profile (v wave cutoff sign).

Alluri N, Kumar S, Marfatia R, et al. Aortic valve **perforation** diagnosed with use of 3-dimensional transesophageal echocardiography. Tex Heart Inst J. 2012;39:590–591.

De Castro S, Cartoni D, d'Amati G, et al. Diagnostic accuracy of transthoracic and multiplane transesophageal echocardiography for valvular **perforation** in acute infective endocarditis: correlation with anatomic findings. Clin Infect Dis. 2000;30:825–826.

Nadji G, Rusinaru D, Remadi JP, et al. **Heart failure** in left-sided native valve infective endocarditis: characteristics, prognosis, and results of surgical treatment. Eur J Heart Fail. 2009;11:668–675.

Tribouilloy C, Rusinaru D, Sorel C, et al. Clinical characteristics and outcome of infective endocarditis in adults with **bicuspid** aortic valves: a multicentre observational study. Heart. 2010;96:1723–1729.

ENDOCARDITIS OF IMPLANTED ELECTRONIC DEVICES

- The rate of cardiac device infections is increasing.
- Endocarditis of a pacemaker requires *extraction* of the entire pacing system.
- A mobile echodensity attached to a pacemaker wire may be a thrombus, a fibrin strand, or a vegetation.
- Clinical judgment must be used. For example, a mass without positive blood cultures, or other evidence of infection, is more likely to represent a thrombus.

Athan E, Chu VH, Tattevin P, et al. Clinical characteristics and outcome of infective endocarditis involving implantable cardiac **devices**. JAMA. 2012;307:1727–1735.

Victor F, De Place C, Camus C, et al. **Pacemaker** lead infection: echocardiographic features, management, and outcome. Heart. 1999;81:82–87.

Baddour LM, Epstein AE, Erickson CC, et al. Update on cardiovascular implantable electronic device infections and their management: a scientific statement from the American Heart Association. Circulation. 2010;121:458–477.

This guideline explains biofilm. Echo is useful for diagnosing complications: endocarditis of right and left cardiac valves, septic pulmonary emboli, mycotic pulmonary artery aneurysm.

Marrie TJ, Costerton JW. Morphology of **bacterial attachment** to cardiac pacemaker leads and power packs. J Clin Microbiol. 1984;19:911–914.

Electron microscope images of biofilm.

NONBACTERIAL THROMBOTIC ENDOCARDITIS

- Valvular vegetations can be *sterile*.
- They are associated with certain conditions:
  - Metastatic malignancies: Adenocarcinomas of the lung, pancreas, or gastrointestinal tract.
  - Systemic lupus erythematosus: Libman-Sacks endocarditis.

Eiken PW, Edwards WD, Tazelaar HD, et al. **Surgical pathology** of nonbacterial thrombotic endocarditis in 30 patients, 1985–2000. Mayo Clin Proc. 2001;76:1204–1212.

Nonbacterial thrombotic endocarditis (NBTE) in a surgical population was more commonly associated with autoimmune disorders than malignancy or disseminated intravascular coagulopathy. Women were affected twice as often as men. Systemic embolization, particularly to the brain, was prominent in both surgical and autopsy series. Vegetations had a similar appearance regardless of the specific underlying disease. An antemortem diagnosis of NBTE in a patient with no known risk factors should prompt a search not only for occult malignancy, as suggested by autopsy studies, but also for autoimmune or rheumatic diseases, particularly the antiphospholipid syndrome.

el-Shami K, Griffiths E, Streiff M. Nonbacterial thrombotic endocarditis in **cancer** patients: pathogenesis, diagnosis, and treatment. Oncologist. 2007;12:518–523.

NBTE is a serious and potentially underdiagnosed manifestation of a prothrombotic state that can cause substantial morbidity in affected patients, most notably recurrent or multiple ischemic cerebrovascular strokes. Diagnosis of NBTE requires a high degree of clinical suspicion as well as the judicious use of two-dimensional echocardiography to document the presence of valvular thrombi. In the absence of contraindications to therapy, treatment consists of systemic anticoagulation, which may ameliorate symptoms and prevent further thromboembolic episodes, as well as control of the underlying malignancy whenever possible.

Silbiger JJ. The cardiac manifestations of **antiphospholipid syndrome** and their echocardiographic recognition. J Am Soc Echocardiogr. 2009;22:1100–1108.

Silbiger JJ. The valvulopathy of non-bacterial thrombotic endocarditis. J Heart Valve Dis. 2009;18:159–166.

BLOOD CYSTS

- These are congenital, thin-walled valve leaflet cysts filled with non-organized (unclotted) blood. The size ranges from microscopic to an echocardiographically visible 0.3 cm. Occasionally they are larger, or multiple.
- Blood cysts are rarely diagnosed in an adult echo lab. They are a well-known incidental finding during infant autopsies.
- However, the diagnosis of a possible blood cyst should be entertained in the differential diagnosis of *every* patient with a suspected vegetation.
- In other words, *every* echocardiographer should be familiar with this typically benign valve leaflet finding that should not be mistaken for a vegetation.
- True echocardiographers think of a blood cyst every time they accidentally bite down on their own cheek.

Agac MT, Acar Z, Turan T, et al. Blood cyst of **tricuspid** valve: an incidental finding in a patient with ventricular septal defect. Eur J Echocardiogr. 2009;10:588–589.

Dencker M, Jexmark T, Hansen F, et al. Bileaflet blood cysts on the **mitral** valve in an adult. J Am Soc Echocardiogr. 2009;22:1085.

Gallucci V, Stritoni P, Fasoli G, et al. Giant blood cyst of **tricuspid** valve. Successful excision in an infant. Br Heart J. 1976;38:990–992.

López-Pardo F, López-Haldón J, Granado-Sánchez C, et al. A heart inside the heart: blood cyst of **mitral** valve. Echocardiography. 2008;25:928–930.

Park MH, Jung SY, Youn HJ, et al. Blood cyst of subvalvular apparatus of the **mitral** valve in an adult. J Cardiovasc Ultrasound. 2012;20:146–149.

Paşaoğlu I, Doğan R, Demircin M, et al. Blood cyst of the **pulmonary valve** causing pulmonic valve stenosis. Am J Cardiol. 1993;72:493–494.

Xie SW, Lu OL, Picard MH. Blood cyst of the **mitral** valve: detection by transthoracic and transesophageal echocardiography. J Am Soc Echocardiogr. 1992;5:547–550.

THE DOCTOR AS AN ENDOCARDITIS PATIENT

- The self-observations of a medical student in the journal that he kept until two days before his death from endocarditis at the age of 24 were first published in 1942.

Flegel KM. Subacute bacterial endocarditis observed: the illness of Alfred S. Reinhart. CMAJ. 2002;167:1379–1383.

Korelitz BI. A Harvard medical student chronicles his fatal illness: the story of Alfred S. Reinhart, 1907–1931. Mt Sinai J Med. 1995;62:226–232; discussion 233–234.

VIDEOS

VIDEO 17-1 (A–C). Aortic valve endocarditis.

VIDEO 17-2. Aortic valve endocarditis. Severe aortic regurgitation.

VIDEO 17-3. Bicuspid aortic valve endocarditis.

VIDEO 17-4 (A–C). Aortic prosthesis endocarditis extending to the right atrium.

VIDEO 17-5 (A,B). Fistula from an infected aortic bioprosthesis to the right atrium.

VIDEO 17-6 (A–D). Mitral valve endocarditis.

VIDEO 17-7. "Kissing" mitral valve vegetations.

VIDEO 17-8. Calcified old vegetations on both sides of the posterior mitral leaflet.

VIDEO 17-9. Flail posterior mitral leaflet. No endocarditis.

VIDEO 17-10 (A,B). Tricuspid valve endocarditis.

VIDEO 17-11 (A–C). Mitral bioprosthesis endocarditis.

VIDEO 17-12 (A,B). Partial mitral ring dehiscence. Vegetations on the ring.

VIDEO 17-13 (A,B). Mitral prosthetic ring dehiscence. Severe regurgitation.

VIDEO 17-14 (A–D). Mitral bioprosthesis ring dehiscence.

VIDEO 17-15. Tricuspid bioprosthesis endocarditis.

VIDEO 17-16. Aortic bioprosthesis vegetation.

VIDEO 17-17 (A,B). Aortic root abscess.

VIDEO 17-18 (A,B). Aortic root abscess. Paravalvular and valvular aortic bioprosthesis regurgitation.

VIDEO 17-19. Aortic wall abscess. Thick aortic bioprosthesis leaflets.

VIDEO 17-20. Aortic root abscess—extension to the mitral valve.

VIDEO 17-21. Aortic root abscess. Heart block on ECG.

VIDEO 17-22. Mitral annulus abscess and vegetation.

VIDEO 17-23 (A–D). Aortic bioprosthesis. Aortic root abscess. Fistula to the left atrium.

VIDEO 17-24 (A–F). Pulmonic prosthesis vegetation.

VIDEO 17-25 (A,B). Pulmonic valve endocarditis.

VIDEO 17-26 (A–D). Mitral leaflet perforation.

VIDEO 17-27 (A–D). Perforation of a calcified, previously infected posterior mitral leaflet.

VIDEO 17-28 (A,B). Right atrial wire endocarditis.

VIDEO 17-29 (A,B). Pacemaker wire endocarditis.

VIDEO 17-30. Sidelobe artifact from a nodule of Arantius should not be confused for a vegetation.

VIDEO 17-31 (A,B). Blood cyst.

VIDEO 17-32 (A–C). Mitral bioprosthesis. Papillary muscle stump and flail chordae should not be confused with vegetations.

VIDEO 17-33 (A–D). Chiari network.

VIDEO 17-34. Thin walled Eustachian valve.

VIDEO 17-35 (A,B). Normal nodules of Arantius.

VIDEO 17-36 (A,B). Artifact that crosses anatomic borders and should not be mistaken for a vegetation.

VIDEO 17-37 (A–C). Vegetations are typically larger than the filament like evanescent Lambl excrescences.

Hinton RB, Prakash A, Romp RL, et al. Cardiovascular manifestations of tuberous sclerosis complex and summary of the revised diagnostic criteria and surveillance and management recommendations from the International Tuberous Sclerosis Consensus Group. J Am Heart Assoc. 2014;3:e001493.

Nir A, Tajik AJ, Freeman WK, et al. Tuberous sclerosis and cardiac rhabdomyoma. Am J Cardiol. 1995;76:419–421.

Sciacca P, Giacchi V, Mattia C, et al. Rhabdomyomas and tuberous sclerosis complex: our experience in 33 cases. BMC Cardiovasc Disord. 2014;14:66.

FIBROMA

- Echo appearance: bright echogenic intramyocardial mass. Non-contractile.
- May be confused with localized hypertrophy.
- Pediatric age group.
- Usually solitary.
- Associated with Gorlin syndrome.
- May be associated with malignant arrhythmias.

PHEOCHROMOCYTOMA OF THE HEART

- Typical shape and location:
  - Well circumscribed and ovoid.
  - Located along the atrioventricular groove.
- TEE is used for diagnosis.
- Coronary-supplied blood flow.

Osranek M, Bursi F, Gura GM, et al. Echocardiographic features of pheochromocytoma of the heart. Am J Cardiol. 2003;91:640–643.

HAMARTOMA

- Echo appearance: discrete mass in the ventricular wall with preserved contractility.
- This is a benign collection of disorganized mature cardiac myocytes.

Fealey ME, Edwards WD, Miller DV, et al. Hamartomas of mature cardiac myocytes: report of 7 new cases and review of literature. Hum Pathol. 2008;39:1064–1071.

Mantilla-Hernández JC, Amaya-Mujica J, Alvarez-Ojeda OM. An unusual tumour: hamartoma of mature cardiac myocytes. Rev Esp Patol. 2019;52:50–53.

Raffa GM, Malvindi PG, Settepani F, et al. Hamartoma of mature cardiac myocytes in adults and young: case report and literature review. Int J Cardiol. 2013;163:e28–e30

Raffa GM, Tarelli G, Balzarini L, et al. Hamartoma of mature cardiac myocytes: a cardiac tumour with preserved contractility. Eur Heart J Cardiovasc Imaging. 2013;14:1216.

CARCINOID HEART DISEASE

- Carcinoid tumors are rare, slow-growing neuroendocrine malignancies.
- They originate in the gastrointestinal tract.

TABLE 18-1 • Echocardiographic Features

Tricuspid valve leaflets:
- Thickening.
- Retraction.
- Decreased mobility.
- Loss of leaflet coaptation.
- Severe tricuspid valve regurgitation.
- Right atrial enlargement.
- Right ventricular volume overload.
- Hepatic vein systolic flow reversal.

Pulmonic valve leaflets:
- Thickening.
- Retraction.
- Stenosis.

- They cause no symptoms until they become large or metastasize.
- Carcinoid *syndrome* occurs when tumor cells metastasize to the liver.
- Tumor substances cause flushing, bronchospasm, and diarrhea, and they attack the heart valves.
- Both tricuspid and pulmonary valve leaflets become thickened.
- The right heart is predominantly involved.
- The lungs inactivate the tumor substances (bradykinin and serotonin).
- In 7% there is *left* heart involvement. Lung metastases and/or a patent foramen ovale allow bradykinin and serotonin to reach and damage the left heart valves.
- Metastatic tumor may be embedded in the heart: RV 40%; LV 53%; interventricular septum 7%.
- Carcinoid plaque may be present on the endocardium of the right heart.
- On echo:
  - A combination of valvular regurgitation and stenosis is present.
  - The leaflets become retracted, fixed, and non-coapting.
  - The tricuspid and pulmonic valves remain in a semi-open position.
- Note:
  - Pulmonary stenosis worsens the severity of tricuspid regurgitation.
  - The severity of pulmonary stenosis may be underestimated when there is low cardiac output due to severe tricuspid regurgitation.

Davar J, et al. Diagnosing and managing carcinoid heart disease in patients with neuroendocrine tumors: an **expert statement**. J Am Coll Cardiol. 2017;69:1288–1304.

Hayes AR, Davar J, Caplin ME. Carcinoid heart disease: a **review**. Endocrinol Metab Clin North Am. 2018;47:671–682.

Moller JE, Connolly HM, Rubin J, et al. Factors associated with **progression** of carcinoid heart disease. N Engl J Med. 2003;348:1005–1015.

Omar HR, Mangar D, Fattouch T, et al. **Extracavitary** cardiac carcinoid presenting with right ventricular outflow tract obstruction. Eur Heart J Cardiovasc Imaging. 2015;16:345.

Pandya UH, Pellikka PA, Enriquez-Sarano M, et al. Metastatic carcinoid tumor to the heart: **echocardiographic-pathologic** study of 11 patients. J Am Coll Cardiol. 2002;40:1328–1332.

Pellikka PA, Tajik AJ, Khandheria BK, et al. Carcinoid heart disease: clinical and **echocardiographic** spectrum in 74 patients. Circulation. 1993;87:1188–1196.

Simula DV, Edwards WD, Tazelaar HD, et al. Surgical pathology of carcinoid heart disease: a study of 139 **valves** from 75 patients spanning 20 years. Mayo Clin Proc. 2002;77:139–147.

OTHER CARDIAC TUMORS

Brinckman SL, van der Wouw P. **Angiosarcoma** of the pericardium: a fatal disease. Circulation. 2005;111:e388–e389.

Glancy DL, Roberts WC. The heart in malignant **melanoma**. A study of 70 autopsy cases. Am J Cardiol. 1968;21:555–571.

Kojima S, Sumiyoshi M, Suwa S, et al. Cardiac **hemangioma**: a report of two cases and review of the literature. Heart Vessels. 2003;18:153–156.

Perk G, Yim J, Varkey M, et al. Cardiac cavernous **hemangioma**. J Am Soc Echocardiogr. 2005;18:979.

Thiagaraj A, Kalamkar P, Rahman R, et al. An unprecedented case report of primary cardiac **lymphoma** exclusive to left ventricle: a diagnostic and therapeutic challenge. Eur Heart J Case Rep. 2018;2:yty029.

Tighe DA, Anene CA, Rousou JA, et al. Primary cardiac **lymphoma**. Echocardiography. 2000;17:345–347.

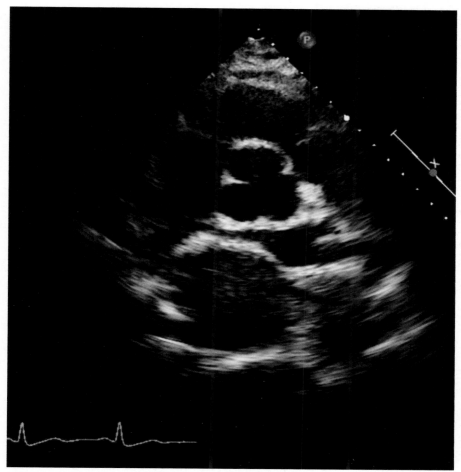

FIGURE 18-3. Hiatus hernia compressing the left atrium.

MIMICS OF CARDIAC TUMORS

- Ultrasound imaging may suggest the presence of a mass in the following examples (Figs. 18-3, 18-4, and 18-5):
  - Prominent Eustachian valve in the right atrium.
  - Prominent ligament of Marshall in the left atrium.
  - Mobile intracardiac thrombus.
  - Large fungal valvular vegetation.

Anfinsen OG, Aaberge L, Geiran O, et al. **Coronary artery aneurysms** mimicking cardiac tumor. Eur J Echocardiogr. 2004;5:308–312.

Cheng HW, Hung KC, Lin FC, Wu D. Spontaneous **intramyocardial hematoma** mimicking a cardiac tumor of the right ventricle. J Am Soc Echocardiogr. 2004;17:394–396.

Choi BJ, Chang HJ, Choi SY, et al. A **coronary artery fistula** with saccular aneurysm mimicking a right atrial cystic mass. Jpn Heart J. 2004;45:697–702.

Chowdhury PS, Timmis SB, Marcovitz PA. Clostridium perfringens within intracardiac thrombus: a case of intracardiac gas **gangrene**. Circulation. 1999;100:2119.

Herbst A, Padilla MT, Prasad AR, et al. Cardiac **Wegener's granulomatosis** masquerading as left atrial myxoma. Ann Thorac Surg. 2003;75:1321–1323.

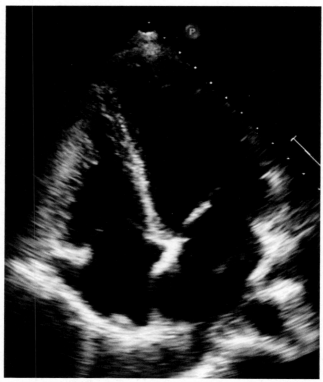

FIGURE 18-4. Normal crista terminalis—a ridge that separates the right atrial appendage from the rest of the right atrial cavity.

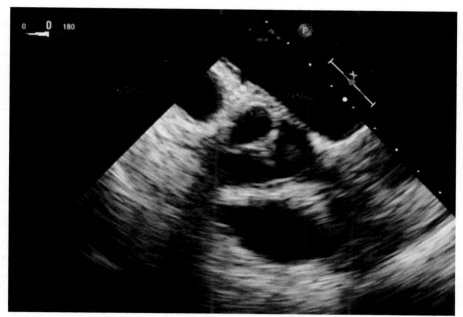

FIGURE 18-5. Tangential cut of a normal left coronary aortic cusp falsely suggesting the presence of a mass.

Ker J, Van Beljon J. **Diaphragmatic hernia** mimicking an atrial mass: a two-dimensional echocardiographic pitfall and a cause of postprandial syncope. Cardiovasc J S Afr. 2004;15:182–183.

Mathew J, Gasior R, Thannoli N. **Fungal mass** on the tricuspid valve. Circulation. 1996;94:2040.

Pappas KD, Arnaoutoglou E, Papadopoulos G. Giant **atrial septal aneurysm** simulating a right atrial tumour. Heart. 2004;90:493.

HYDATID CYST OF THE HEART

- Echinococcosis is a rare parasitic disease.
- It should be considered in patients coming from an endemic area.
- Diagnosis of cardiac hydatid cysts is made with transthoracic echo. TEE provides more details.
- Rupture of a cardiac cyst is a serious complication.
- Imaging is critical for early diagnosis, assessment, and follow-up.

Barbetseas J, Lambrou S, Aggeli C, et al. Cardiac hydatid cysts: echocardiographic findings. J Clin Ultrasound. 2005;33:201–205.

Bouraoui H, Trimeche B, Mahdhaoui A, et al. Echinococcosis of the heart: clinical and echocardiographic features in 12 patients. Acta Cardiol. 2005;60:39–41.

Brunetti E, Tamarozzi F, Macpherson C, et al. Ultrasound and cystic echinococcosis. Ultrasound Int Open. 2018;4:E70–E78.

Thameur H, Abdelmoula S, Chenik S, et al. Cardiopericardial hydatid cysts. World J Surg. 2001;25:58–67.

VIDEOS

VIDEO 18-1 (A–C). Lung cancer with metastasis to the pericardium and right atrium. On initial evaluation, the right atrial tumor was mistakenly diagnosed as a myxoma.

VIDEO 18-2. Lung cancer with metastasis to the heart.

VIDEO 18-3 (A–C). Renal cell carcinoma—metastatic to the right ventricle.

VIDEO 18-4. Renal cell carcinoma extending to the inferior vena cava.

VIDEO 18-5 (A,B). Hypernephroma extending from the kidneys to the right atrium via the inferior vena cava.

VIDEO 18-6 (A–C). Metastatic tumor in the left ventricle.

VIDEO 18-7 (A,B). Lymphoma infiltrating the inferior wall.

VIDEO 18-8 (A–C). Extensive invasion of the heart by lymphoma.

VIDEO 18-9. Melanoma extending to the tricuspid annulus.

VIDEO 18-10 (A–C). Cancer of the esophagus.

VIDEO 18-11 (A,B). External compression of the right heart by a mediastinal mass.

VIDEO 18-12. Left atrial myxoma. Reverberation artifact from the spine.

VIDEO 18-13 (A–E). Left atrial myxoma.

VIDEO 18-14. A highly mobile atrial septal aneurysm may be mistaken for a left atrial mass.

VIDEO 18-15. Atrial septal aneurysm. A tangential cut falsely suggests a left atrial myxoma.

VIDEO 18-16. Mitral annular calcification with calcific nodular protrusions into the left atrial cavity. Dialysis patient.

VIDEO 18-17 (A–F). Right atrial myxoma.

VIDEO 18-18. Pedunculated right atrial tumor attached near the SVC-to-RA junction.

VIDEO 18-19 (A,B). Tumor extending from the superior vena to the right atrium.

VIDEO 18-20. Blood cyst on the left atrial side of the mitral valve.

VIDEO 18-21 (A,B). Papillary fibroelastoma on the left ventricular side of the mitral valve.

VIDEO 18-22. Papillary fibroelastoma on the aortic valve.

VIDEO 18-23 (A–D). Lambl excrescence on the aortic valve.

VIDEO 18-24. Papillary fibroelastoma on the tricuspid valve chordae.

VIDEO 18-25 (A,B). Papillary fibroelastoma on the right ventricular side of the pulmonic valve.

VIDEO 18-26 (A–C). Left ventricular fibroma.

VIDEO 18-27 (A,B). Carcinoid disease of the tricuspid valve.

VIDEO 18-28. Carcinoid disease of the pulmonic valve.

VIDEO 18-29 (A–C). Chiari network is a normal anatomic structure that should not be confused with a right atrial tumor or vegetation.

VIDEO 18-30 (A,B). Patients with end-stage renal failure can develop large mitral annular calcifications in the left atrium that can be confused with tumors.

VIDEO 18-31. Unusually mobile mitral annular calcification in a dialysis patient. Possibly a healed old vegetation. Vegetations usually attach to the leaflet commissure rather than to the annulus.

VIDEO 18-32. Large mitral valve vegetation.

VIDEO 18-33. Caseous mitral annular calcification.

VIDEO 18-34 (A,B). Tangential cut of the left coronary cusp falsely suggests a tumor or a vegetation.

VIDEO 18-35 (A–D). Normal Eustachian valve creating a "shelf" in the right atrium.

VIDEO 18-36 (A–C). Mobile Eustachian valve.

VIDEO 18-37. Large Eustachian valve in the right atrium. Multiple imaging windows were used to confirm the diagnosis.

VIDEO 18-38. Superior vena cava catheter and attached thrombus entering the right atrium.

VIDEO 18-39 (A,B). Right atrial pacemaker wire with an attached thrombus.

VIDEO 18-40. Right ventricular pacemaker wire with an attached thrombus.

VIDEO 18-41. Hiatus hernia: The stomach is interposed between the esophagus and the heart. Note the contrast in the stomach way at the top of the screen. Sipping a carbonated beverage through a straw can confirm this diagnosis.

VIDEO 18-42 (A–C). Reverberation artifact from the tricuspid annulus should not be mistaken for an atrial mass.

VIDEO 18-43. Normal right atrial appendage trabeculations should not be mistaken for a tumor.

VIDEO 18-44. Normal intraventricular structures. The negative contrast should not be mistaken for thrombus or tumor.

VIDEO 18-45. Prominent crista terminalis that should not be mistaken for a right atrial tumor. Unrelated findings: Posterior mitral leaflet prolapse, descending thoracic aorta next to the left atrial free wall.

VIDEO 18-46. Crista terminalis.

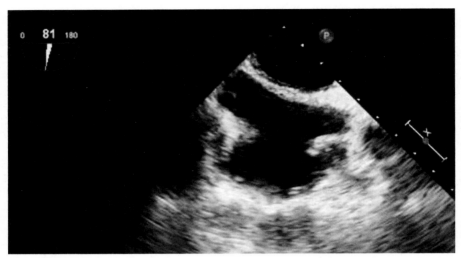

FIGURE 18-6. Crista terminalis.

VIDEO 18-47. Coiled right atrial pacemaker wire can be mistaken for a right atrial mass.

VIDEO 18-48. Lipomatous atrial septal hypertrophy.

VIDEO 18-49. Lipomatous atrial septal hypertrophy extending around to the crista terminalis.

VIDEO 18-50 (A–C). Lipomatous atrial septal hypertrophy with edge enhancement and reverberation artifacts.

VIDEO 18-51. Intrapericardial fibrin may not be distinguishable from an intrapericardial tumor.

VIDEO 18-52. Normal tricuspid papillary muscle should not be mistaken for a tumor.

VIDEO 18-53. Calcified papillary muscle tips.

VIDEO 18-54. Reverberation and attenuation caused by a right ventricular catheter.

VIDEO 18-55. Reverberation artifact from a false tendon.

VIDEO 18-56 (A,B). Range ambiguity: A late reflection returning from far past the heart can confuse the ultrasound machine electronics. It gets interpreted as a reflection coming from a later ultrasound pulse. The image of the reflection is wrongly placed closer to the transducer.

VIDEO 18-57. Multiple reverberation artifacts at the tissue–blood interface.

VIDEO 18-58. Hiatus hernia by the left ventricular apex.

VIDEO 18-59. Hiatus hernia. Patient is sipping soda through a straw while images are being acquired.

VIDEO 18-60. Thrombus in the descending aorta. Patient had heparin-induced thrombocytopenia.

CHAPTER 19

Diabetes and Hypertension

DIABETES MELLITUS

- Metabolic syndrome:
  - Elevated fasting glucose.
  - Elevated blood pressure.
  - Elevated waist circumference.
  - Elevated triglycerides.
  - Reduced high-density lipoprotein cholesterol.
- Echo in a diabetic may reveal wall motion abnormalities of a previously undiagnosed silent myocardial infarction.
- Diabetics with coronary artery disease may be referred for complete revascularization with bypass surgery, rather than partial revascularization with a stent.
- Echo assessment of left ventricular systolic and diastolic function, as well as a search for regional left ventricular wall motion abnormalities, may help in this decision.

Ernande L, Bergerot C, Girerd N, et al. Longitudinal myocardial **strain** alteration is associated with left ventricular remodeling in asymptomatic patients with type 2 diabetes mellitus. J Am Soc Echocardiogr. 2014;27:479–488.

Hare JL, Hordern MD, Leano R, et al. Application of an exercise intervention on the evolution of **diastolic dysfunction** in patients with diabetes mellitus: efficacy and effectiveness. Circ Heart Fail. 2011;4:441–449.

Hwang YC, Jee JF, Kang M, et al. Metabolic syndrome and insulin resistance are associated with abnormal left ventricular **diastolic function** and structure independent of blood pressure and fasting plasma glucose level. Int J Cardiol. 2012;159:107–111.

Kosmala W, Przewlocka-Kosmala M, Wojnalowicz A, et al. **Integrated backscatter** as a fibrosis marker in the metabolic syndrome: association with biochemical evidence of fibrosis and left ventricular dysfunction. Eur Heart J Cardiovasc Imaging. 2012;13:459–467.

Seferović PM, Paulus WJ. Clinical diabetic **cardiomyopathy**: a two-faced disease with restrictive and dilated phenotypes. Eur Heart J. 2015;36:1718–1727.

Shindler DM, Kostis JB, Yusuf S, et al. Diabetes mellitus, a predictor of morbidity and **mortality** in the Studies of Left Ventricular Dysfunction (SOLVD) Trials and Registry. Am J Cardiol. 1996;77:1017–1020.

Zoroufian A, Razmi T, Taghavi-Shavazi M, et al. Evaluation of subclinical left ventricular dysfunction in diabetic patients: longitudinal strain velocities and left ventricular dyssynchrony by two-dimensional **speckle tracking** echocardiography study. Echocardiography. 2014;31:456–463.

HYPERTENSIVE HEART DISEASE

> ### GUIDELINES
>
> *Marwick TH, Gillebert TC, Aurigemma G, et al. Recommendations on the use of echocardiography in adult hypertension. Eur Heart J Cardiovasc Imaging. 2015;16:577–605.*
>
> - Normal values for left ventricular mass.
> - Echocardiographic calculation of left ventricular mass.
> - Left ventricular geometric patterns.
> - Imaging of myocardial fibrosis.

- Left ventricular hypertrophy (LVH) is used clinically as an indicator of cardiac end-organ damage due to hypertension.
- It is important for the sonographer to learn to identify the classic unmistakable ECG of LVH.
- Once LVH develops on the ECG, it is a *permanent* marker of hypertensive heart disease.
- Treatment of hypertension may favorably affect the extent of LVH.
- It is possible to compare available sequential echo studies to look for changes in LVH.
- M-mode calculation of LV mass had been used extensively in the past as a simple measure of *reversibility*.
- Pitfall: The calculated M-mode changes in LV mass are valid only if the left ventricle is not dilated due to associated valvular disease, and there are no aneurysms or other geometry-distorting LV wall motion abnormalities. A sigmoid septum (septal "knuckle" due to basal septal hypertrophy), commonly found in older patients, also may affect this measurement.
- Diastolic function can be affected by long-standing untreated hypertension. It may be manifested as dyspnea that progresses to heart failure with preserved ejection fraction (HFpEF).
- A reduced E/A ratio of mitral valve inflow (A>E) is commonly found in severely hypertensive young patients. It is easy to perform. (Pulsed-wave Doppler interrogation should be at the mitral leaflet tips.)
- It is most useful for identifying diastolic dysfunction in younger hypertensives. It is found with advancing age in normotensive patients.
- Tissue Doppler and myocardial strain offer more sophisticated parameters of left ventricular systolic and diastolic dysfunction, but they may not distinguish hypertensive heart disease from other cardiomyopathies.
- E/e' ratio can estimate left atrial pressures and can help guide diuretic treatment of hypertension and dyspnea. An atrial (S4) gallop may be heard on cardiac auscultation and can subsequently disappear when symptoms improve with treatment. Serial auscultation is less expensive than serial echocardiograms.

- Left atrial enlargement and mitral regurgitation also may be present in hypertensive heart disease.
- When the aorta becomes affected by hypertension, it may become aneurysmal.
- Aortic regurgitation may result from dilatation of the sinuses of Valsalva.

Campens L, Demulier L, De Groote K, et al. **Reference values** for echocardiographic assessment of the diameter of the aortic root and ascending aorta spanning all age categories. Am J Cardiol. 2014;114:914–920.

Mirea O, Maffessanti F, Gripari P, et al. Effects of aging and body size on proximal and ascending aorta and aortic arch: inner edge **reference values** in a large adult population by two-dimensional transthoracic echocardiography. J Am Soc Echocardiog. 2013;26:419–427.

Law of Laplace

- Practical illustration of wall tension in a hypertensive left ventricle, and in a hypertensive aorta: Pressure = wall tension ÷ radius
- A partially inflated, sausage-shaped *toy balloon* illustrates the following:
  - The balloon feels "firm" where the radius is the greatest (aorta).
  - The balloon feels "soft" at the nipple where the radius is small (left ventricle).
  - Yet the pressure inside the entire balloon is the same!
  - Systolic pressure is the same in the left ventricle and in the aorta (when there is no aortic stenosis).
  - A progressively dilating aorta may eventually rupture because of increased wall tension.
  - A small *hypertrophic* hypertensive left ventricle strives to maintain a small radius to reduce wall tension.

Bang CN, Gerdts E, Aurigemma GP, et al. **Four-group classification** of left ventricular hypertrophy based on ventricular concentricity and dilatation identifies a low-risk subset of eccentric hypertrophy in hypertensive patients. Circ Cardiovasc Imaging. 2014;7:422–429.

de Simone G, Izzo R, Aurigemma GP, et al. Cardiovascular risk in relation to a new **classification** of hypertensive left ventricular geometric abnormalities. J Hypertens. 2015;33:745–754.

Santos M, Shah AM. Alterations in **cardiac structure** and function in hypertension. Curr Hypertens Rep. 2014;16:428.

Preoperative Clearance in Hypertension

- Dobutamine stress echo is frequently performed for preoperative clearance in patients with end-stage renal disease.
- Uncontrolled hypertension may affect interpretation.
- Left ventricular cavity obliteration at peak stress may cause hypotension without underlying ischemia.
- A frequently asked question is whether it is safe to perform dobutamine stress echocardiography on a patient with marked aneurysmal distention of the abdominal aorta.

Pellikka PA, Roger VL, Oh JK, et al. **Safety** of performing dobutamine stress echocardiography in patients with abdominal aortic aneurysm > or = 4 cm in diameter. Am J Cardiol. 1996;77:413–416.

*Ninety-eight patients with abdominal aortic aneurysms ≥4 cm in diameter were identified. Records were reviewed to determine whether there was any evidence of aneurysm rupture or adverse vascular events as a result of the stress test. There was **no case of aneurysm rupture** or hemodynamic instability precipitated by dobutamine stress echocardiography. In addition, dobutamine stress echocardiography that was negative for ischemia **identified patients at very low risk** of perioperative cardiac events.*

Preoperative Considerations in Valvular Regurgitation

- Severe valvular stenosis, pulmonary hypertension, unstable angina, heart failure, and malignant arrhythmias increase perioperative risk.
- Many anesthetic regimens *reduce afterload*, so both mitral and aortic regurgitation may hemodynamically improve during anesthesia.
- When comparing aortic regurgitation and mitral regurgitation, there is a difference when it comes to afterload: The severity of both lesions is affected by changes in preload, but aortic regurgitation is affected more significantly by changes in afterload.
- The best way to understand this is to first review what happens in diastole.
- Diastolic filling is affected both in mitral regurgitation and in aortic regurgitation:
  - In mitral regurgitation diastolic filling is affected by the increased filling from the distended and overfilled left atrium.
  - In aortic regurgitation diastolic filling is affected by continuous filling from the aorta into the left ventricle.
  - In aortic regurgitation, during diastole, the severity of the regurgitation will determine the degree of filling of the left ventricle.
  - In systole, the left ventricle in the patient with aortic regurgitation has to eject into an aorta that was not designed to accommodate the amount of stroke volume created by severe aortic regurgitation.
- In contrast, the left ventricle in the patient with mitral regurgitation "ejects" into the low-impedance left atrium at the same time that it ejects into the aorta.
- Echocardiographic corollary: The presence of severe left ventricular *dilatation* is a useful marker of hemodynamically significant aortic regurgitation. As opposed to mitral regurgitation, progressive left ventricular dilatation does not beget more aortic regurgitation. If the left ventricle is becoming progressively dilated, the aortic regurgitation can be held responsible.
- Imaging pitfall: The color flow display of mitral regurgitation in the left atrium *does* change dramatically with changes in afterload, because it reflects the left ventricular driving pressure (systolic blood pressure). The color flow area of mitral regurgitation also decreases dramatically after a stenotic aortic valve is replaced.

- There is normal respiratory "lung sliding"—the pleural line moves with respiration.
- In patients with heart failure and increased extravascular lung water, there may be *vertical* (instead of horizontal) reverberation artifacts at the pleural line.
- Lung ultrasound is effective at detecting a pneumothorax:
  - There is a pleural line on ultrasound, but no evident "lung sliding" due to air between the visceral and parietal pleura.
  - The usual pleural reverberation artifacts are absent.
  - The edge of a pneumothorax is identified at the transition point from normal "lung sliding" to a pleural line without "lung sliding."
  - Lung ultrasound may help decide whether thoracentesis is required in some patients, and it can subsequently help in guiding this procedure.
  - Unrecognized one-lung intubations (also known as main-stem intubation) can lead to hypoventilation, atelectasis, barotrauma, and even death. Bilateral lung sliding can confirm proper endotracheal intubation, especially among patients with cardiac arrest.

Gargani L, Volpicelli G. How I do it: lung ultrasound. Cardiovascular Ultrasound. 2014;12:25.

Llamas-Alvarez AM, Tenza-Lozano EM, Latour-Perez J. Accuracy of lung ultrasonography in the diagnosis of **pneumonia** in adults: systematic review and meta-analysis. Chest. 2017;151:374–382.

Pivetta E, et al. Lung ultrasound-implemented diagnosis of acute decompensated **heart failure** in the ED: a SIMEU multi-center study. Chest. 2015;148:202–210.

Rose G, Siadecki S, Tansek R, et al. A novel method of assessing for **lung sliding** using Doppler imaging. Am J Emerg Med. 2017;35:1738–1742.

Sim SS, Lien WC, Chou HC, et al. Ultrasonographic lung sliding sign in confirming proper **endotracheal intubation** during emergency intubation. Resuscitation. 2012;83:307–312.

Williamson JP, Grainge C, Parameswaran A, et al. **Thoracic ultrasound**: what non-radiologists need to know. Curr Pulmonol Rep. 2017;6:39–47.

PLATYPNEA AND ORTHODEOXIA

- Platypnea is dyspnea in the upright position.
- It is the converse of orthopnea.
- Platypnea is relieved by assuming the recumbent position.
- Orthodeoxia is arterial desaturation in the upright position.
- Echo is used to look for a patent foramen ovale, and for a pericardial effusion.
- If a patent foramen is discovered, echo is used to look for a postural increase in right-to-left shunting in the sitting position.
- A *pericardial effusion* can distort the right atrial architecture in the standing position.
- In these patients, there may be right-to-left shunting in the standing position.

Acharya SS, Kartan R. A case of orthodeoxia caused by an **atrial septal aneurysm**. Chest. 2000;118:871–874.

Faller M, Kessler R, Chaouat A, et al. Platypnea-orthodeoxia syndrome related to an **aortic aneurysm** combined with an aneurysm of the atrial septum. Chest. 2000;118:553–557.

*Ferry TG, Naum CC. Orthodeoxia-platypnea due to **diabetic** autonomic neuropathy. Diabetes Care. 1999;22:857–859.*

*Kennedy TC, Knudson RJ. Exercise-aggravated hypoxemia and orthodeoxia in **cirrhosis**. Chest. 1977;72:305–309.*

ASTHMA

- Patients with asthma may be referred by a pulmonologist for an echo.
- Churg-Strauss is a rare syndrome that presents with asthma and can have echocardiographic findings related to vasculitis.
- Patients with hypereosinophilic syndrome can have apical left ventricular thrombi.

*Eroglu E, Di Salvo G, Herbots L, et al. Restrictive left ventricular filling in **hypereosinophilic** syndrome as a result of partial cavity obliteration by an apical mass: a strain/strain rate study. J Am Soc Echocardiogr. 2003;16:1088–1090.*

*Morgan JM, Raposo L, Gibson DG. Cardiac involvement in **Churg-Strauss** syndrome shown by echocardiography. Br Heart J. 1989;62:462–466.*

*Ommen SR, Seward JB, Tajik AJ. Clinical and echocardiographic features of **hypereosinophilic** syndromes. Am J Cardiol. 2000;86:110–113.*

*Pelà G, Tirabassi G, Pattoneri P, et al. Cardiac involvement in the **Churg-Strauss** syndrome. Am J Cardiol. 2006;97: 1519–1524.*

*Sen T, Gungor O, Akpinar I, et al. Cardiac involvement in **hypereosinophilic** syndrome. Tex Heart Inst J. 2009;36:628–629.*

VIDEOS

VIDEO 20-1 (A–D). Artifact from ultrasound-facilitated thrombolysis of pulmonary embolism.

VIDEO 20-2. Erroneous assignment of color to some reverberation artifacts. The ultrasound system assumes that tissue moves slowly and blood moves quickly. Slow-moving ultrasound signals are depicted in grayscale. Rapidly moving signals are assigned a color.

VIDEO 20-3 (A–E). McConnell sign in pulmonary embolism.

VIDEO 20-4. Mobile thrombus in the inferior vena cava.

VIDEO 20-5. Slice thickness artifact: Fibrin from a pleural effusion wrongly suggests an intracardiac mass.

VIDEO 20-6 (A,B). Mirror image artifact should not be mistaken for a pleural effusion.

VIDEO 20-7. Right-to-left atrial septal displacement.

VIDEO 20-8. TAPSE: normal longitudinal right ventricular systolic function.

VIDEO 20-9. Normal right atrial pressure. Normal decrease of inferior vena cava diameter with a sniff.

VIDEO 20-10. Dilated inferior vena cava.

VIDEO 20-11. Catheter entering the right atrium from the inferior vena cava.

VIDEO 20-12. A large left pleural effusion can create an acoustic window to the heart. The images of the heart were obtained from the back with the transducer positioned next to the left scapula.

VIDEO 20-13. Lung ultrasound—comet tail reverberation artifacts.

VIDEO 20-14. Right pleural effusion that may be mistaken for a loculated pericardial effusion.

VIDEO 20-15. Right pleural effusion.

VIDEO 20-16 (A–C). Fibrin in the pleural space.

VIDEO 20-17. TEE is superior to TTE for imaging catheters in the superior vena cava.

VIDEO 20-18 (A,B). Rapid pulmonary artery flow acceleration and mid-systolic slowing in pulmonary hypertension.

VIDEO 20-19. Pleural fluid "sliding" across the pericardium.

VIDEO 20-20 (A,B). Severe tricuspid regurgitation and pulmonary hypertension. Contrast reversal into the hepatic veins.

VIDEO 20-21. Normal right ventricular moderator band.

VIDEO 20-22 (A–D). Right ventricular trabeculations.

VIDEO 20-23. Biventricular hypertrophy.

VIDEO 20-24. Normal right ventricular free wall longitudinal strain.

VIDEO 20-25. Pulmonary hypertension. Left ventricular strain.

VIDEO 20-26. Subjectively decreased longitudinal systolic contraction of the anterior right ventricular wall.

VIDEO 20-27. Normal short-axis right ventricular dimensions and function.

VIDEO 20-28. Subcostal view of the pulmonic valve.

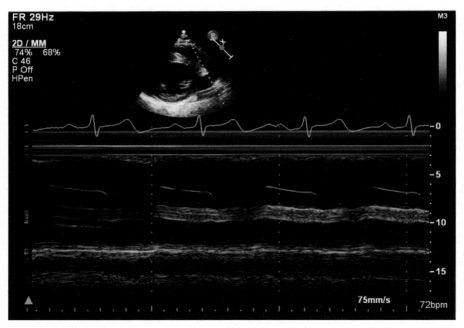

FIGURE 20-4. Absent pulmonic valve A wave in pulmonary hypertension.

VIDEO 20-29. Dilated hypokinetic right ventricle.

VIDEO 20-30 (A,B). Right ventricular pressure overload. The interventricular septum stays flat in systole.

VIDEO 20-31. Pulmonary hypertension. Systolic and diastolic septal flattening. Dilated right ventricle.

VIDEO 20-32 (A,B). Right ventricular volume overload. The left ventricle assumes a round shape in systole.

VIDEO 20-33 (A,B). Combined right ventricular pressure and volume overload. The left ventricle attempts to assume a round shape in systole.

VIDEO 20-34 (A,B). Right ventricular hypertrophy. Prominent right ventricular trabeculations.

VIDEO 20-35. Pulmonary hypertension. Right ventricular hypertrophy. Right-to-left atrial septal displacement.

VIDEO 20-36. Pulmonary hypertension. Right ventricular dilatation and hypertrophy. Right-to-left atrial septal displacement.

VIDEO 20-37. Pulmonary hypertension. Patent foramen ovale.

VIDEO 20-38. Abnormal right ventricular strain.

VIDEO 20-39. Right ventricular infarction. Abnormal right ventricular strain.

VIDEO 20-40. Apical right ventricular thrombus.

VIDEO 20-41. Pacemaker wire—tricuspid leaflet retraction.

VIDEO 20-42. Normal caval inflow into the right atrium.

VIDEO 20-43. Inferior vena cava blood directed toward the heart in blue. Brief flow reversal in red.

VIDEO 20-44. Left upper and left lower pulmonary veins.

VIDEO 20-45. Dilated pulmonary artery.

VIDEO 20-46. Two separate pulmonic regurgitation jets.

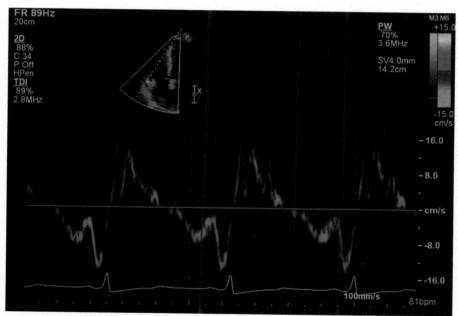

FIGURE 20-5. Tricuspid annulus tissue Doppler.

VIDEO 20-47. Moderate pulmonic valve regurgitation in a patient with diastolic pulmonary hypertension.

VIDEO 20-48. Pericardial effusion and pulmonary hypertension.

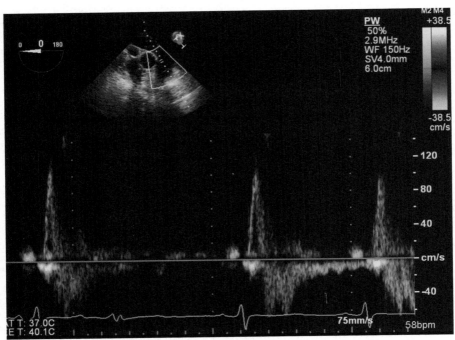

FIGURE 20-6. Increased pulmonary vascular resistance.

VIDEO 20-49 (A–C). Spontaneous contrast in the inferior vena cava.

VIDEO 20-50. Normal respiratory variation of inferior vena cava diameter.

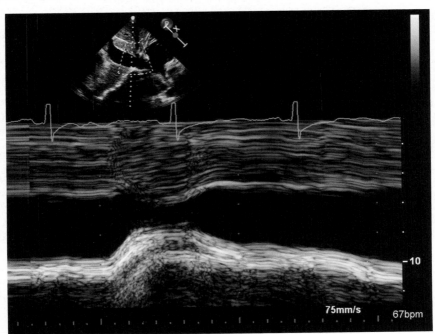

FIGURE 20-7. Normal respiratory variation of inferior vena cava diameter.

VIDEO 20-51 (A,B). Cardiac compression by pectus excavatum.

VIDEO 20-52. Respiratory attenuation of ultrasound by the lung.

VIDEO 20-53. Imaging the heart through a pleural effusion. The transducer is located below the left scapula.

VIDEO 20-54. Motion of fibrinous pleural fluid discordant to cardiac motion.

VIDEO 20-55. Normal fractional area change of the right ventricular outflow.

NOTES

CHAPTER 21

Tricuspid Valve

GUIDELINES

Huttin O, Voilliot D, Mandry D, et al. All you need to know about the tricuspid valve: tricuspid valve imaging and tricuspid **regurgitation analysis**. Arch Cardiovasc Dis. 2016;109:67–80.

Zoghbi WA, Adams D, Bonow RO, et al. Recommendations for noninvasive evaluation of native valvular regurgitation. J Am Soc Echocardiogr. 2017;30:303–371.

Table 14 and images show the echocardiographic determination of tricuspid regurgitation severity.

ANATOMY

"The tricuspid valve is septophylic. The mitral valve is septophobic."

- Tricuspid chordae can insert directly into the interventricular septum. Mitral chordae do not. This can help distinguish the tricuspid valve from the mitral valve when imaging congenital disorders.
- The normal tricuspid annulus is saddle shaped.
- There are anterior, posterior, and septal tricuspid valve leaflets.
- An estimated 80% of significant tricuspid regurgitation is functional.
- Functional tricuspid regurgitation is due to distortion of:
    - Right ventricular size.
    - Tricuspid annulus geometry.
    - Tricuspid support apparatus.
- As functional tricuspid regurgitation gets worse, the tricuspid annulus dilates, becomes *flatter*, and becomes more circular.

Acar C, Périer P, Fontaliran F, et al. **Anatomical study** of the tricuspid valve and its variations. Surg Radiol Anat. 1990;12: 229–230.

Anwar AM, Geleijnse ML, Soliman OI, et al. Assessment of normal tricuspid valve **anatomy** in adults by real-time three-dimensional echocardiography. Int J Cardiovasc Imaging. 2007;23:717–724.

Badano LP, Agricola E, Perez de Isla L, et al. Evaluation of the tricuspid valve morphology and function by transthoracic real-time **three-dimensional** echocardiography. Eur J Echocardiogr. 2009;10:477–484.

Dreyfus GD, Martin RP, Chan KM, et al. **Functional** tricuspid regurgitation: a need to revise our understanding. J Am Coll Cardiol. 2015;65:2331–2336.

Fukuda S, Gillinov AM, Song JM, et al. Echocardiographic insights into atrial and ventricular **mechanisms** of functional tricuspid regurgitation. Am Heart J. 2006;152:1208–1214.

Fukuda S, Saracino G, Matsumura Y, et al. Three-dimensional geometry of the **tricuspid annulus** in healthy subjects and in patients with functional tricuspid regurgitation: a real-time, 3-dimensional echocardiographic study. Circulation. 2006;114:1492–1498.

A staging system for functional tricuspid valve pathology using three parameters:

- Tricuspid regurgitation severity.
- Annular dilation.
- Mode of leaflet coaptation (extent of tethering).

Ton-Nu TT, Levine RA, Handschumacher MD, et al. **Geometric determinants** of functional tricuspid regurgitation: insights from 3-dimensional echocardiography. Circulation. 2006;114:143–149.

TRICUSPID VALVE TRAUMA AND CHORDAL RUPTURE

- Tricuspid regurgitation can be caused by blunt chest trauma or by endomyocardial biopsy.
- Tricuspid valves can be involved in 20% of *myxomatous* mitral valve disease. There can be prolapse, elongation of chordae, and rare chordal rupture.
- Significant pacemaker lead–induced tricuspid regurgitation is associated with a poor prognosis.

Al-Mohaissen MA, Chan KL. Prevalence and mechanism of tricuspid regurgitation following implantation of endocardial leads for **pacemaker** or cardioverter-defibrillator. J Am Soc Echocardiogr. 2012;25:245–252.

Braverman AC, Coplen SE, Mudge GH, et al. Ruptured chordae tendineae of the tricuspid valve as a complication of **endomyocardial biopsy** in heart transplant patients. Am J Cardiol. 1990;66:111–113.

Chiu WC, Shindler DM, Scholz PM, et al. Traumatic tricuspid regurgitation with **cyanosis**: diagnosis by transesophageal echocardiography. Ann Thorac Surg. 1996;61:992–993.

Emine BS, Murat A, Mehmet B, et al. Flail mitral and tricuspid valves due to **myxomatous** disease. Eur J Echocardiogr. 2008;9:304–305.

Hoke U, Auger D, Thijssen J, et al. Significant lead-induced tricuspid regurgitation is associated with poor prognosis at long-term follow-up. Heart. 2014;100:960–968.

Kim JB, Spevack DM, Tunick PA, et al. The effect of transvenous pacemaker and implantable cardioverter defibrillator **lead placement** on tricuspid valve function: an observational study. J Am Soc Echocardiogr. 2008;21:284–287.

Kleikamp G, Schnepper U, Körtke H, et al. Tricuspid valve regurgitation following blunt thoracic **trauma**. Chest. 1992;102:1294–1296.

Weinreich DJ, Burke JF, Bharati S, et al. Isolated **prolapse** of the tricuspid valve. J Am Coll Cardiol. 1985;6:475–481.

RIGHT HEART ENDOCARDITIS

- Congenital heart disease can predispose patients to right heart endocarditis.
- There was a 43% prevalence of asymptomatic mitral valve prolapse in a predominantly addicted population of 51 patients with tricuspid valvular endocarditis caused by *Staphylococcus aureus*.

- Patients may present with pulmonary manifestations: cough, hemoptysis, pleuritic pain, pulmonary embolism, pleural effusions, pneumonia, pulmonary infarct, abscess, and empyema.
- Removal of the tricuspid valve without valve replacement has been done occasionally to control the infection in intravenous heroin addicts in whom the valve has been destroyed by infectious endocarditis.
- Imaging notes:
  - Transesophageal imaging of right heart endocarditis is not necessarily superior and should be combined with transthoracic imaging.
  - Because of their generally larger size (compared with mitral and aortic valve vegetations), tricuspid valve vegetations may remain on the valve after bacteriologic cure.
  - Vegetations >2.0 cm are associated with increased mortality.

Arbulu A, Holmes RJ, Asfaw I. Tricuspid valvulectomy without replacement. Twenty years' experience. J Thorac Cardiovasc Surg. 1991;102:917–922.

Bayer AS, Blomquist IK, Bello E, et al. Tricuspid valve endocarditis due to Staphylococcus aureus. Correlation of two-dimensional echocardiography with clinical outcome. Chest. 1988;93:247–253.

Hecht SR, Berger M. Right-sided endocarditis in intravenous drug users. Prognostic features in 102 episodes. Ann Intern Med. 1992;117:560–566.

Hust MH, Metzler B, Ebermann F, et al. Tricuspid valvulectomy in antibiotic-refractory right-heart endocarditis. Dtsch Med Wochenschr. 1997;122:80–85.

Macedo J, Grawe ES. Hypoxemia requiring venovenous extracorporeal membrane oxygenation after tricuspid valvulectomy for infective endocarditis. CASE (Phila). 2019;3:183–186.

Panidis IP, Kotler MN, Mintz GS, et al. Clinical and echocardiographic correlations in right heart endocarditis. Int J Cardiol. 1984;6:17–34.

Of 23 patients, 20 (87%) had a history of intravenous drug abuse.

van der Westhuizen NG, Rose AG. Right-sided valvular infective endocarditis. A clinicopathological study of 29 patients. S Afr Med J. 1987;71:25–27.

EBSTEIN ANOMALY

"Apical tethering and abnormal attachment of the tricuspid leaflets to the endocardial surface of the right ventricle."

- During normal embryologic development, the tricuspid leaflets grow by separating away from the embryonic right ventricular walls. This is called *delamination*.
- In Ebstein anomaly, there is some degree of failure of separation of the tricuspid leaflets from this embryonic myocardium.
- The severity of the disorder is variable.
- Severe forms of the disorder are more common in neonates.
- Some newborns may have massive cardiomegaly.
- Another subset of newborns may present with severe cyanosis for several days after birth. The cyanosis slowly decreases as neonatal pulmonary vascular resistance continues to drop, and pulmonary blood flow can consequently

increase. The cause of the temporary cyanosis is a right-to-left shunt across a commonly associated atrial septal defect.

- In the most severe Ebstein cases, echo may show no mobile tricuspid valve tissue.
- Adult Ebstein patients have variable degrees of:
  - Apical tethering of the tricuspid leaflets, and apical displacement of their hinge points.
  - The septal and posterior leaflet motion is restricted.
  - The functional valve orifice becomes apically displaced.
  - The anterior leaflet appears sail-like and larger than normal, domes in diastole, and moves like a whip.
  - The closure of the anterior leaflet is delayed, and the leaflet is visualized in the RVOT in PLAX.
  - Simply put, Ebstein anomaly is an exaggeration of the normal, more apical tricuspid valve attachment. In reality, it is a complex disorder with an extensive spectrum of variable manifestations.
  - On echo: The septal insertion point of the tricuspid valve is compared with the septal insertion of the anterior mitral leaflet.
  - Diagnosis: The distance between the mitral and tricuspid insertion points can be divided by the patient's body surface area.
  - A displacement index >8 mm/m^2 is diagnostic for Ebstein anomaly.
  - In the adult, apical tricuspid displacement of ≥20 mm also is used for diagnosis.
  - The displacement index helps differentiate Ebstein anomaly from tricuspid valve dysplasia.
  - In tricuspid dysplasia there is no apical hinge point displacement. Chordae are short. Leaflets are thickened. There are gaps in systolic leaflet coaptation that create tricuspid regurgitation.
- Echo is used to:
  - Establish the diagnosis.
  - Determine the degree of tricuspid regurgitation (less frequently, degree of tricuspid stenosis).
  - Evaluate right ventricular size and function (Fig. 21-1).
  - If the functional area of the right ventricle is less than one-third of the total right ventricle, the prognosis is poor.
  - Look for associated abnormalities: right ventricular outflow obstruction by the large anterior tricuspid leaflet, atrial septal defect, patent foramen ovale, pulmonic valve stenosis.
  - Employ this information to guide possible surgical repair.
  - After surgical repair, echo is used to follow the function of the repaired tricuspid valve.
  - Ebstein patients may have left ventricular dysfunction. This is associated with a poor prognosis.
  - Surgical repair makes use of systolic anterior leaflet contact with interventricular septum, creating a functioning monocusp valve.

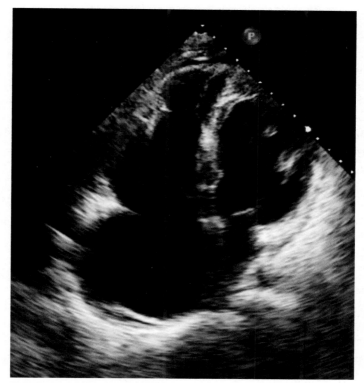

FIGURE 21-1. Ebstein anomaly.

- Alternatively, the newer *cone procedure* mobilizes the anterior and posterior tricuspid valve leaflets from their abnormal attachment points. The free edge of this leaflet complex is rotated clockwise and sutured to the septal border of the anterior leaflet. This creates a cone. The vertex is fixed at the right ventricular apex. The base is sutured to the normal tricuspid annulus plane.

Attenhofer Jost CH, Connolly HM, Dearani JA, et al. Ebstein's anomaly. Circulation. 2007;115:277–285.

Excellent review.

Rodés-Cabau J, Taramasso M, O'Gara PT. Diagnosis and treatment of tricuspid valve disease: current and future perspectives. Lancet. 2016;388:2431–2442.

AUSCULTATION AND ECHO IN TRICUSPID REGURGITATION

"Color flow Doppler reliably detects all degrees of tricuspid regurgitation—except perhaps when you need it most: when it is wide open."

- The size of the color flow jet is the starting point for determining tricuspid regurgitation severity. Bedside physical examination is equally important.
- Other echocardiographic measures and findings include:
  - Doppler characteristics such as signal strength and signal duration.

- Contour by continuous wave may show early systolic deceleration and late systolic cutoff.
- PISA and vena contracta determine regurgitant volume.
- Increased right atrial and right ventricular size should be noted.
- The shape of the interventricular septum helps to differentiate between severe right ventricular *pressure* overload and severe right ventricular *volume* overload.
- Loss of leaflet coaptation can be demonstrated with 2D echo.
- Leaflet thickening and retraction are found in *carcinoid* tricuspid valve disease.
- Chordal rupture can occur with trauma.
- Leaflet destruction may be seen with endocarditis.
- Pacemaker wires and catheters across the tricuspid valve cause variable degrees of regurgitation. 3D imaging should always be used.
- Bedside examination after the echocardiographic diagnosis is useful for follow-up decisions.
- The neck vein findings may be influenced by pericardial compliance.
- An increase in the loudness of the tricuspid regurgitation murmur during inspiration is a classic finding.
- The Doppler tricuspid regurgitation signal also increases during respiration.
- The following *bedside auscultation technique* may be useful to evaluate a murmur for respiratory variation:
  - Inspiration may be too distracting to comment on the change in loudness of the tricuspid regurgitation murmur.
  - During held deep expiration, left-sided murmurs should become *more* audible because there is less interposed air between the stethoscope and the heart.
  - During held deep expiration, tricuspid regurgitation becomes *less* audible.

Brickner PW, Scudder WT, Weinrib M. Pulsating varicose veins in functional tricuspid insufficiency. Case report and venous pressure tracing. Circulation. 1962;25:126–129.

As the degree of cardiac compensation improves, the physical signs of tricuspid insufficiency disappear.

Hansing CE, Rowe GG. Tricuspid insufficiency. A study of hemodynamics and pathogenesis. Circulation. 1972;45:793–799.

Duroziez described a xiphoid systolic murmur, enlarged right atrium, distended neck veins with systolic pulsation, hepatic enlargement and pulsation, and peripheral cyanosis.

The characteristic murmur with its inspiratory accentuation may be missed even in cases with severe tricuspid insufficiency.

Jugular venous V waves are not always present and may be obscured by distended neck veins.

The hepatic pulsation is readily detected only with severe tricuspid insufficiency and may be confused with a transmitted pulse from the aorta or right ventricle.

The severity of tricuspid insufficiency is influenced by exercise, deep breathing, and cardiac function.

Hultgren HN. Venous pistol shot sounds. Am J Cardiol. 1962;10:667–672.

Morgan JR, Forker AD. Isolated tricuspid insufficiency. Circulation. 1971;43:559–564.

*A useful test is the **Valsalva** maneuver; the murmur of tricuspid insufficiency will return in about 1 s on release of Valsalva, whereas left heart murmurs will usually not return for 3 s or longer.*

Muller O, Shillingford J. Tricuspid incompetence. Br Heart J. 1954;16:195–207.

Detailed description of the murmur.

Topilsky Y, Tribouilloy C, Michelena HI, et al. Pathophysiology of tricuspid regurgitation: quantitative Doppler echocardiographic assessment of **respiratory** dependence. Circulation. 2010;122:1505–1513.

Verel D, Sandler G, Mazurkie SJ. Tricuspid incompetence in cor pulmonale. Br Heart J. 1962;24:441–444.

In patients with emphysema, cor pulmonale, or rheumatic heart disease, the site of maximal intensity of the tricuspid insufficiency murmur is commonly over the free edge of the liver.

TRICUSPID STENOSIS

- The most common cause of tricuspid stenosis in an adult in our lab is a malfunctioning tricuspid prosthesis.
- Only 3% to 5% of patients with rheumatic mitral valve disease have associated tricuspid stenosis.
- The accepted pressure half time for a tricuspid stenosis area of 1 cm^2 is 190 ms.
- A mean diastolic gradient of 5 mm Hg or more indicates severe tricuspid stenosis.
- Measurements should be scrutinized for respiratory changes.

Bousvaros GA, Stubington D. Some auscultatory and phonocardiographic features of tricuspid stenosis. Circulation. 1964;29:26–33.

Fawzy ME, Mercer EN, Dunn B, et al. Doppler echocardiography in the evaluation of tricuspid stenosis. Eur Heart J. 1989;10:985–990.

Kitchin A, Turner R. Diagnosis and treatment of tricuspid stenosis. Br Heart J. 1964;26:354–379.

Rivero-Carvallo JM. El diagnostico de la estenosis tricuspidea. Arch Inst Cardiol Mexico. 1950;20:1.

VIDEOS

VIDEO 21-1. Short-axis view of the tricuspid valve.

VIDEO 21-2. Normal attachment of tricuspid septal leaflet chordae to the interventricular septum.

VIDEO 21-3. Anterior, septal, and posterior leaflets of the tricuspid valve.

VIDEO 21-4. Tricuspid papillary muscle.

VIDEO 21-5. The normal tricuspid valve is apically displaced in relation to the mitral valve. Ebstein abnormality is an "exaggeration of normal."

VIDEO 21-6 (A,B). Absent longitudinal excursion of the tricuspid annulus.

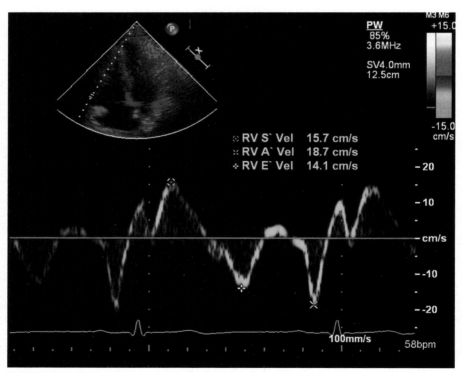

FIGURE 21-2. Tissue Doppler of the tricuspid annulus.

VIDEO 21-7. Severe tricuspid regurgitation.

VIDEO 21-8. Severe tricuspid regurgitation. The pacemaker wire appears to limit the closing motion of the anterior tricuspid leaflet.

VIDEO 21-9. Severe tricuspid regurgitation due to loss of leaflet coaptation. Dilated right atrium and right ventricle.

VIDEO 21-10. Short duration of pulmonic regurgitation. Elevated right ventricular end-diastolic pressure.

VIDEO 21-11 (A–C). Hepatic vein systolic flow reversal. Severe tricuspid regurgitation.

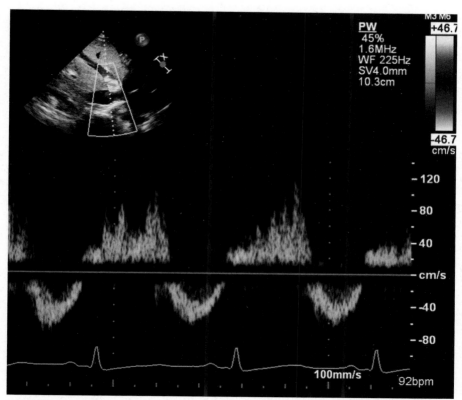

FIGURE 21-3. Hepatic vein systolic flow reversal. Severe tricuspid regurgitation.

VIDEO 21-12. Saline contrast reversal into a hepatic vein. Severe tricuspid regurgitation.

VIDEO 21-13 (A–E). Loss of tricuspid leaflet coaptation.

VIDEO 21-14. Tricuspid regurgitation and aortic leaflet opening can be used to time systole. Caval inflow is both systolic and diastolic.

VIDEO 21-15. Normal tricuspid valve anatomy.

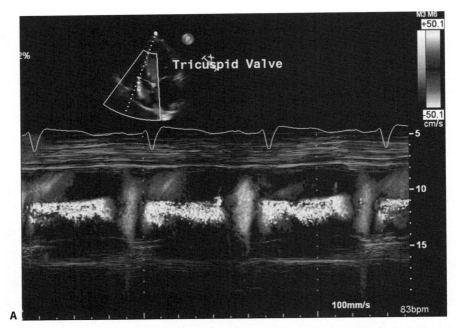

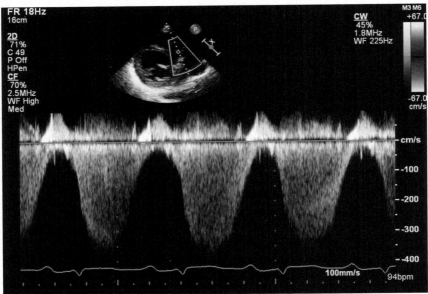

FIGURE 21-4 (A,B). Tricuspid regurgitation that starts in the isovolumic period, continues through systole and into diastole, stopping after the atrial contraction.

CHAPTER 22

Pulmonic Valve

PULMONIC VALVE REGURGITATION

- Mild degrees of pulmonic valve regurgitation are common in normal individuals. This should be considered a normal variant.
- The regurgitant color flow jets may be eccentric.
- Scanning tip: Timing the jet with pulsed-wave Doppler, or with color M-mode Doppler, will help distinguish it from coronary artery flow and from a continuous communication between the aorta and the pulmonary artery.
- Note: Severe pulmonic valve regurgitation with normal pulmonary pressures may be of short duration and may have a low velocity.
- The guidelines integrate magnetic resonance imaging with echocardiography for quantitation of PR. This is particularly important in patients with congenital heart disease.
- Significant pulmonic valve regurgitation may be:
  - An indicator of pulmonary diastolic hypertension.
  - A consequence of pulmonary valve endocarditis.
  - A sign of a bicuspid, quadricuspid, absent, or dysplastic pulmonic valve.
  - Associated with a dilated pulmonary artery.
  - Important in prior tetralogy repair.
  - An indicator of a failing pulmonic homograft in a Ross procedure.
  - Present in carcinoid pulmonic valve disease.
- Findings in severe pulmonary valve regurgitation:
  - Jet width to RVOT ratio ≥70%.
  - Pressure half time <100 ms.
  - Early jet termination.
  - Premature pulmonic valve opening.
  - Pulmonary artery diastolic flow reversal.

Dellas C, Kammerer L, Gravenhorst V, et al. Quantification of pulmonary regurgitation and prediction of pulmonary valve replacement by echocardiography in patients with **congenital heart defects** in comparison to cardiac magnetic resonance imaging. Int J Cardiovasc Imaging. 2018;34:607–613.

*Fathallah M, Krasuski RA. Pulmonic valve disease: review of **pathology** and current treatment options. Curr Cardiol Rep. 2017;19:108.*

*Fernández-Armenta J, Villagómez D, Fernández-Vivancos C, et al. **Quadricuspid** pulmonary valve identified by transthoracic echocardiography. Echocardiography. 2009;26:288–290.*

*Renella P, Aboulhosn J, Lohan DG, et al. Two-dimensional and Doppler echocardiography reliably predict **severe** pulmonary regurgitation as quantified by cardiac magnetic resonance. J Am Soc Echocardiogr. 2010;23:880–886.*

*Takao S, Miyatake K, Izumi S, et al. Clinical implications of pulmonary regurgitation in **healthy** individuals: detection by cross sectional pulsed Doppler echocardiography. Br Heart J. 1988;59:542–550.*

*Waller BF, Howard J, Fess S. **Pathology** of pulmonic valve stenosis and pure regurgitation. Clin Cardiol. 1995;18:45–50.*

PULMONIC VALVE STENOSIS

- Valve opening:
  - In pulmonic valve stenosis, the atrial contraction will open the stenotic valve a crack in late diastole, and it will then remain open until the end of systole, closing at the beginning of next diastole.
  - The reason is that in isolated valvular pulmonic stenosis, the right ventricle becomes muscular and stiff but does not dilate.
  - Atrial contraction elevates the pressure in this noncompliant right ventricle above the relatively low pulmonary artery diastolic pressure, and the valve opens and stays ajar.
  - The appearance of partly open stenotic pulmonic leaflets is fused leaflets that dome with a circular orifice—like a short windsock, or the mouth of a volcano.
- Auscultation:
  - The ejection click of valvular pulmonic stenosis is an exception to the useful clinical rule that right-sided murmurs increase on inspiration.
- The loudness of an ejection click is determined by the distance the pulmonic valve travels before stopping short with a resulting click.
- On inspiration the right heart fills more because of the negative intrathoracic pressure.
- A doming stenotic pulmonic valve travels *less* during inspiration than it does when the heart is smaller in expiration.
- Examining the patient during *held expiration* will also make the ejection click more audible.
  - The loudness of the systolic pulmonic stenosis murmur correlates with severity.
  - It may be harsh and sound like someone is clearing their throat.
  - It may radiate to the back.
- Imaging pitfalls:
  - The right ventricle becomes dilated in patients with atrial septal defects, not in patients with isolated valvular pulmonic stenosis.
  - It is a common echocardiographic misinterpretation that patients with dilated right heart chambers due to an atrial septal defect have pulmonic stenosis. The increased blood flow in the pulmonary artery from the shunt increases the systolic Doppler flow velocities.

- Tricuspid regurgitation velocity indicates right ventricular "driving" pressure—in other words, the pressure gradient between the right ventricle and the right atrium in systole. The velocity increases in pulmonic stenosis and may be misinterpreted as pulmonary hypertension.
- The right ventricular systolic pressure is equal to the pulmonary artery systolic pressure *plus* the pulmonary stenosis gradient.
- In pulmonic stenosis patients with an associated restrictive ventricular septal defect, the Doppler velocity indicates the interventricular gradient. As the right ventricular pressure rises in worsening pulmonic stenosis, the velocity of the ventricular septal defect decreases.

Bruce CJ, Connolly HM. Right-sided valve disease deserves a little more respect. Circulation. 2009;119:2726–2734.

NOTES

CHAPTER 23

Disorders of the Aorta

GUIDELINES

*Boodhwani M, Andelfinger G, Leipsic J. **Canadian** Cardiovascular Society position statement on the management of thoracic aortic disease. Can J Cardiol. 2014;30:577–589.*

Erbel R, Aboyans V, Boileau C. 2014 ESC Guidelines on the diagnosis and treatment of aortic diseases: document covering acute and chronic aortic diseases of the thoracic and abdominal aorta of the adult. Eur Heart J. 2014;35:2873–2926.

- Extensive document with mention of rare disorders.
- Genetic diseases that affect the aorta.
- Coral reef aorta.
- Aortic tumors.

*Goldstein SA, Evangelista A, Abbara S, et al. Multimodality **imaging** of diseases of the thoracic aorta in adults. J Am Soc Echocardiogr. 2015;28:119–182.*

- Normal dimensions of the aorta.
- Echo measurement of the proximal ascending aorta.
- Images of dissection.
- Aortic regurgitation in dissection.
- Imaging of intramural hematomas and penetrating aortic ulcers.
- Imaging in coarctation.

*Hiratzka LF, Bakris GL, Beckman JA, et al. **2010 guidelines** for the diagnosis and management of patients with thoracic aortic disease. J Am Coll Cardiol. 2010;55:e27–e129.*

AORTIC DISSECTION

- Diagnosis of dissection:
  - The availability of CT scanning in emergency departments has now made CT a more common *initial* imaging mode than TEE.
  - TEE is still used to rapidly diagnose dissection in critically ill patients who are too unstable to be placed in a CT scanner.

- TEE is used instead of CT in patients where renal dysfunction prohibits the use of contrast for the CT images.
- Local physician expertise also may influence the use of CT versus TEE for initial diagnosis.
- When the diagnosis is made on CT, TEE will still be subsequently used in patients intraoperatively during the repair.
- Transthoracic echo is useful only for initial diagnosis in those rare instances when an intimal flap is clearly visualized.
- Both TTE and TEE can detect and evaluate the consequences of dissection:
  - Pericardial effusion. (The mode of death in this lethal disorder is most commonly cardiac tamponade.)
  - Aortic regurgitation. (It may be possible to save the aortic valve by resuspending it during repair of the dissection.)
  - If the dissection extends to a coronary ostium, the dissection can cause myocardial infarction. In that case, there may be left ventricular wall motion abnormalities on echo associated with ECG abnormalities of infarction.

Imaging

- Numerous artifacts can be present in the proximal ascending aorta, making the confident diagnosis of a dissection flap difficult on PLAX TTE (Fig 23-1).

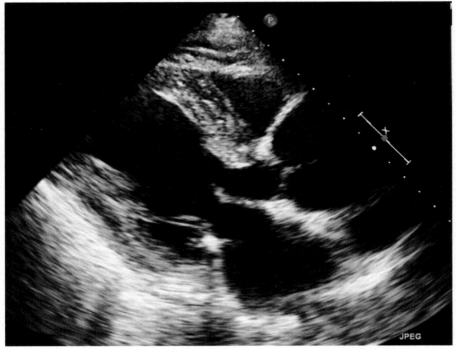

FIGURE 23-1. Annuloaortic ectasia in Marfan syndrome. There is pear-shaped aneurysmal dilatation of the proximal ascending aorta. There is no narrowing of the aorta at the junction between the sinus of Valsalva and the ascending aorta (sinotubular junction).

MITRAL REGURGITATION ON ECHO IN PATIENTS WITH AORTIC DISSECTION

- Understanding the mechanism of mitral regurgitation helps the surgeon decide whether to leave it alone during emergency surgical repair of a dissection.
- New mitral regurgitation following aortic dissection may be due to:
  - New aortic valve regurgitation → left ventricular dilatation → mitral annular dilatation.
  - Coronary ostial occlusion from the dissection → left ventricular wall motion abnormalities → papillary muscle dysfunction.
- Chronic mitral regurgitation in a patient with aortic dissection may be due to:
  - Left ventricular hypertrophy due to long standing hypertension → mitral regurgitation.
  - Marfan syndrome → mitral valve prolapse.

Chiu P, Irons M, van de Rijn M, et al. Giant **pulmonary artery** aneurysm in a patient with Marfan syndrome and pulmonary hypertension. Circulation. 2016;133:1218–1221.

Lim MH, Je HG, Lee SK. Minimally invasive mitral valve repair in a woman with Marfan syndrome and type B dissection. Korean J Thorac Cardiovasc Surg. 2018;51:61–63.

Mazzucotelli JP, Deleuze PH, Baufreton C, et al. Preservation of the aortic valve in acute aortic dissection: long-term echocardiographic assessment and clinical outcome. Ann Thorac Surg. 1993;55:1513–1517.

VIDEOS

VIDEO 23-1 (A–C). Aortic arch.

VIDEO 23-2. Normal proximal ascending aorta.

VIDEO 23-3. Artifact in the proximal ascending aorta that can be confused with a dissection flap.

VIDEO 23-4. Artifact over the descending aorta that can be confused with a dissection flap.

VIDEO 23-5. Arc-shaped sidelobe artifact over the descending aorta that can be confused with a dissection flap.

VIDEO 23-6 (A,B). Descending aorta adjacent to the spine.

VIDEO 23-7. Descending aorta behind the left atrium.

VIDEO 23-8. Aneurysm and dissection flap in the descending aorta behind the heart.

VIDEO 23-9. Descending aorta from the subcostal window.

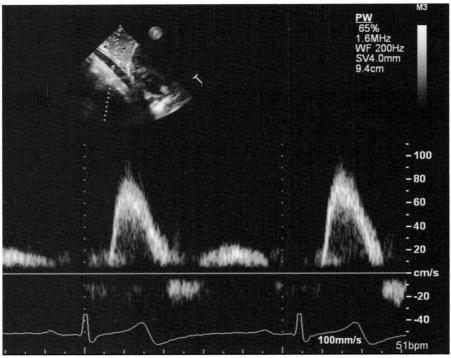

FIGURE 23-4. Descending aorta from the subcostal window.

VIDEO 23-10. Saline contrast in the azygous vein.

VIDEO 23-11. Normal aortic arch and adjacent innominate vein. This should not be misdiagnosed as a dissection.

VIDEO 23-12. Spontaneous contrast in a normal innominate vein. This should not be misdiagnosed as a false lumen of a dissection.

VIDEO 23-13. Sidelobe artifact originating at the aortic leaflet closure. It should not be mistaken for a dissection flap.

VIDEO 23-14. Dissection flap near the aortic valve.

VIDEO 23-15. Dissection flap near the aortic valve. Aortic valve regurgitation.

VIDEO 23-16. Dissection flap in the proximal ascending aorta.

VIDEO 23-17. Dissection of the proximal ascending aorta. Triangular delineation of pericardial effusion in the transverse sinus.

VIDEO 23-18 (A,B). Dissection of the proximal ascending aorta.

VIDEO 23-19. Dissection flap in the proximal ascending aorta slightly above the aortic leaflets.

VIDEO 23-20. Dissection flap in the proximal ascending aorta slightly above the aortic leaflets. Mild aneurysmal dilatation of the aorta.

VIDEO 23-21. Dissection flap near the aortic valve. Reverberation artifact in the descending aorta.

VIDEO 23-22. Dissection flap in the aortic arch.

VIDEO 23-23 (A–D). Dissection flap in the descending aorta.

VIDEO 23-24. Dissection flap in the descending aorta. Spontaneous contrast in the false lumen.

VIDEO 23-25. Dissection flap in the descending aorta. Small true lumen.

VIDEO 23-26. Dissection flap in the descending aorta. Mirror image artifact.

VIDEO 23-27 (A,B). Dissection. False lumen depressurizing into the true lumen in diastole.

VIDEO 23-28. Communication between the true and the false lumen.

VIDEO 23-29. Reverberation artifact from the sinus of Valsalva.

VIDEO 23-30 (A,B). Normal innominate vein flow next to the aortic arch. No dissection.

VIDEO 23-31. Systolic forward flow in the proximal ascending aorta with diastolic flow reversal that generates coronary artery perfusion.

VIDEO 23-32 (A–E). Large atheroma in the descending thoracic aorta.

VIDEO 23-33. Aortic atheroma. Reverberation artifacts in the pleural space.

VIDEO 23-34 (A,B). Dissection of the descending aorta beginning at the left subclavian artery.

VIDEO 23-35 (A,B). Dissection flap in the descending aorta. Subcostal window.

VIDEO 23-36. Intramural hematoma.

VIDEO 23-37. Reverberation artifact in the descending aorta. No dissection.

VIDEO 23-38. Pleural effusion adjacent to a mildly atherosclerotic aorta.

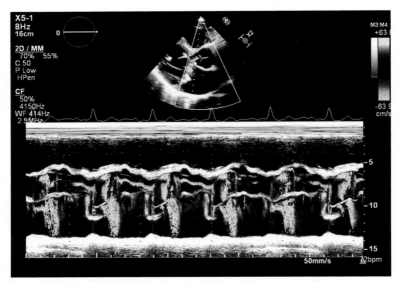

FIGURE 23-5. Think of Marfan syndrome when there is aortic regurgitation and mitral valve prolapse.

VIDEO 23-39 (A,B). Annuloaortic ectasia. Pear-shaped aneurysmal proximal ascending thoracic aorta in a patient with Marfan syndrome.

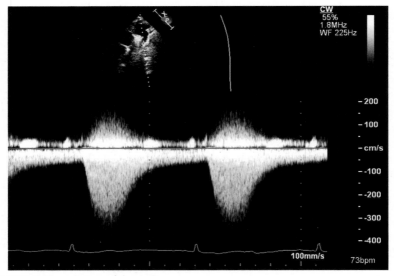

FIGURE 23-6. Coarctation of the aorta.

VIDEO 23-40 (A,B). Coarctation of the aorta.

VIDEO 23-41. Subtle, easily missed, curved, 2D reflection from the wall of a sinus of Valsalva aneurysm protruding into the right ventricular outflow.

VIDEO 23-42 (A–E). Sinus of Valsalva aneurysm.

VIDEO 23-43. Aneurysm of the right sinus of Valsalva.

VIDEO 23-44 (A,B). Sinus of Valsalva aneurysm outlined by color Doppler in the right ventricular outflow.

VIDEO 23-45 (A,B). The ascending aorta should not be mistaken for a right atrium.

VIDEO 23-46. Left atrial compression by a large thrombosed aneurysm of the descending thoracic aorta.

VIDEO 23-47. Left atrial compression by scoliosis.

VIDEO 23-48. Normal curved outline of spine vertebra behind the left atrium.

VIDEO 23-49. Descending aorta branch flow.

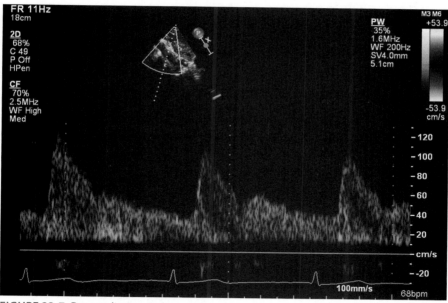

FIGURE 23-7. Descending aorta branch flow.

CHAPTER 24

Stroke

GUIDELINES

Celeste F, Muratori M, Mapelli M, et al. The evolving role and use of echocardiography in the evaluation of cardiac source of embolism. J Cardiovasc Echogr. 2017;27:33–44.

Pepi M, Evangelista A, Nihoyannopoulos P, et al. Recommendations for echocardiography use in the diagnosis and management of cardiac sources of embolism. Eur J Echocardiogr. 2010;11: 461–476.

European Guidelines

- Detailed recommendations for the use of echocardiography.
- Potential cardioembolic sources.
- Echocardiographic predictors of embolic risk.

Saric M, Armour AC, Arnaout MS, et al. Guidelines for the use of echocardiography in the evaluation of a cardiac source of embolism. J Am Soc Echocardiogr. 2016;29:1–42.

- Comprehensive, very readable guideline document that discusses all causes of cardioembolic strokes.
- There are extensive, practical discussions of endocarditis as a source of embolism, embolism from the aorta, cardiac tumors as a source of embolism, and paradoxical and pulmonary embolism, as well as left ventricular and left atrial abnormalities.

ECHO FOR CARDIAC SOURCE OF EMBOLISM

- Role of echo:
  - Establish the existence of a potential cardiac source of embolism (intracardiac thrombus, vegetation, aortic atheroma, interatrial communication, left atrial myxoma).
  - Help determine the likelihood that a stroke came from this source.

Example

- A patient with a mitral or aortic valve vegetation has a stroke, and the vegetation is now clearly smaller in size compared with an echo before the stroke.

- This suggests that part of the vegetation broke off and embolized to the brain.
- Both TTE and TEE imaging are employed.
- TTE is better for confirming an apical left ventricular thrombus.
- Findings on TTE may suggest a potential cardiac source of embolism and may require TEE for confirmation.
- TEE is better for diagnosing:
  - Thrombus in the left atrial appendage.
  - Imaging Tip: See Figures 24-1 to 24-5 for examples of stroke-related TEE information about the left atrial appendage. The challenge for the sonographer is to reproduce some of these TEE findings on transthoracic imaging. This requires creating high resolution 2D and 3D transthoracic images of the left atrial appendage. Imaging angle should also be adjusted with the help of color Doppler so that the pulsed wave Doppler sample volume at the mouth of the appendage is as parallel to blood flow as possible.
  - Atheromas in the aorta—usually found by TEE in the descending thoracic aorta and aortic arch (far less frequently confirmed by TEE in the ascending aorta).
  - Patent foramen ovale—visualized on TEE, but saline contrast with cough and Valsalva also should be done with TTE.
  - Vegetations—better detail on TEE. TEE exam has to be meticulous. Can be missed on TTE.
- TEE is likely to help after TTE if:
  - TTE images are suboptimal.

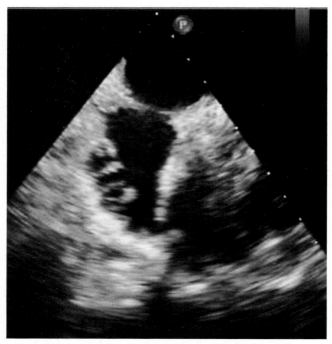

FIGURE 24-1. Prominent left atrial appendage trabeculations.

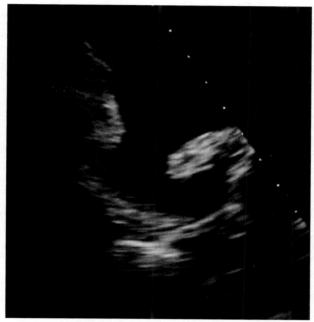

FIGURE 24-2. Sharply angled "chicken wing" left atrial appendage.

- Patient is young, has no previous cardiac condition, and PFO is suspected.
- Prosthetic valve is present.
- Atrial fibrillation is known or suspected.
- Mitral stenosis is present (suspect an LAA thrombus).

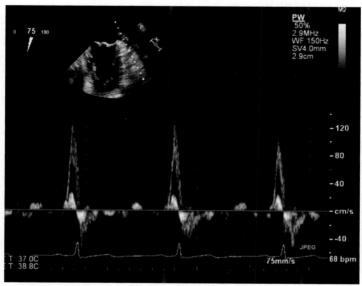

FIGURE 24-3. Rapid emptying velocity of the left atrial appendage after the atrial contraction.

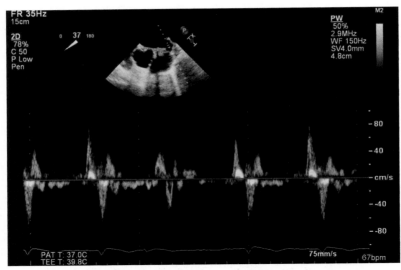

FIGURE 24-4. Normal left atrial appendage velocities.

- Mobile masses on an aortic valve that can embolize:
  - Vegetation.
  - Lambl excrescence—small fibrin strand, 1 or 2 mm in thickness.
  - Papillary fibroelastoma—shimmering, bigger than a Lambl, around 3 mm diameter (or bigger) echodensity attached to an aortic leaflet commissure by a stalk.
- Anatomic structures on the aortic valve that do not embolize:
  - Nodules of Arantius.
  - Raphe on a bicuspid aortic valve.
  - Aortic valve fenestrations (difficult to image).

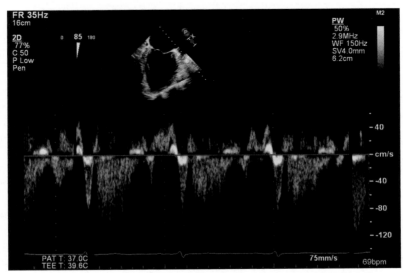

FIGURE 24-5. Mitral regurgitation in the left atrial appendage should reduce the chance of thrombus formation.

VIDEOS

VIDEO 24-1 (A–C). Triangular left atrial appendage.

VIDEO 24-2. Sharply angled left atrial appendage. Prominent trabeculations. No thrombus.

VIDEO 24-3 (A,B). Sharply angled left atrial appendage.

VIDEO 24-4 (A–F). Left atrial appendage thrombus.

VIDEO 24-5. Mural left atrial appendage thrombus despite seemingly normal left atrial appendage contraction.

VIDEO 24-6 (A,B). Dense spontaneous contrast in the left atrial appendage.

VIDEO 24-7 (A–D). Normal left atrial appendage trabeculations (pectinate muscles). No thrombus.

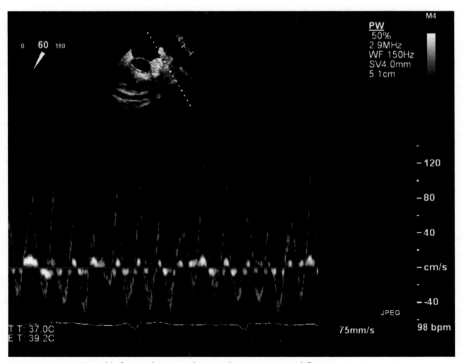

FIGURE 24-6. Rapid left atrial appendage velocities in atrial flutter.

VIDEO 24-8. Incomplete suture closure of the left atrial appendage during open heart surgery.

VIDEO 24-9. Beam width artifact. Fibrin in the pericardial space of the transverse sinus that surrounds the left atrial appendage—appears wrongly to be inside the left atrial appendage.

VIDEO 24-10 (A,B). Reverberation artifact in the left atrial appendage.

VIDEO 24-11. Attenuation artifact in the left atrial appendage.

VIDEO 24-12 (A,B). Left atrial thrombus that originates in the left atrial appendage.

VIDEO 24-13 (A,B). Normal prominent left atrial appendage tissue fold that should not be mistaken for a mass.

VIDEO 24-14 (A–D). Patent foramen ovale—positive saline contrast study.

VIDEO 24-15. Patent foramen ovale—positive saline contrast study. Right-to-left atrial septal displacement.

VIDEO 24-16. Patent foramen ovale. Biatrial enlargement.

VIDEO 24-17 (A,B). Left to right color flow across a foramen ovale.

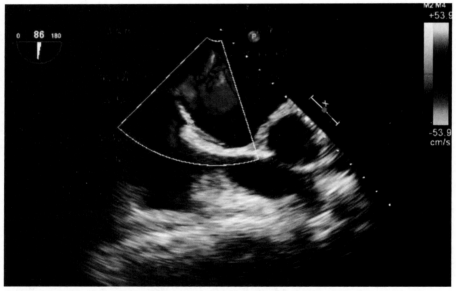

FIGURE 24-7. Left to right color flow across a foramen ovale.

VIDEO 24-18 (A–C). Iatrogenic atrial septal fenestration following Watchman device insertion. Sinus rhythm.

VIDEO 24-19 (A,B). Patent foramen ovale anatomy. Increased flow across the foramen when snoring.

VIDEO 24-20. Thrombus in transit across a patent foramen ovale.

VIDEO 24-21. Bicaval TEE view of the membrane of the fossa ovalis.

VIDEO 24-22. Bicaval view from the subcostal window. A catheter is entering the right atrium from the inferior vena cava.

VIDEO 24-23 (A–C). Patent foramen ovale on TEE.

VIDEO 24-24. Patent foramen ovale. Biatrial enlargement.

VIDEO 24-25 (A,B). Right atrial pacemaker wires.

VIDEO 24-26. Right ventricular pacemaker wire.

VIDEO 24-27. Biventricular pacing. Right atrial pacemaker directed toward the coronary sinus.

VIDEO 24-28 (A–G). Atrial septal aneurysm.

VIDEO 24-29. Atrial septal aneurysm and patent foramen ovale.

VIDEO 24-30 (A,B). Atrial septal aneurysm. Amyloid cardiomyopathy.

VIDEO 24-31 (A,B). Rapid motion of the atrial septum in atrial flutter.

VIDEO 24-32 (A,B). Rapid motion of the left atrial appendage in atrial flutter.

VIDEO 24-33. Atrial fibrillation. Dilated left atrium.

VIDEO 24-34. Patent foramen ovale flow and superior vena cava flow.

VIDEO 24-35 (A,B). Pacemaker wire across the tricuspid valve.

VIDEO 24-36 (A–G). Watchman closure device deployed in the left atrial appendage.

VIDEO 24-37 (A–C). Watchman device: residual communication between the appendage and the left atrial cavity.

VIDEO 24-38. Spontaneous contrast in the superior vena cava. Atrial fibrillation.

VIDEO 24-39. Transpulmonary saline contrast shunt entering the left atrium via a left pulmonary vein.

VIDEO 24-40. Papillary muscles in dilated cardiomyopathy. Not thrombi, because of the mid-ventricular location.

VIDEO 24-41. Lambl excrescences are usually considered incidental findings in stroke patients. However, they must then be distinguished echocardiographically from vegetations, and from papillary fibroelastomas.

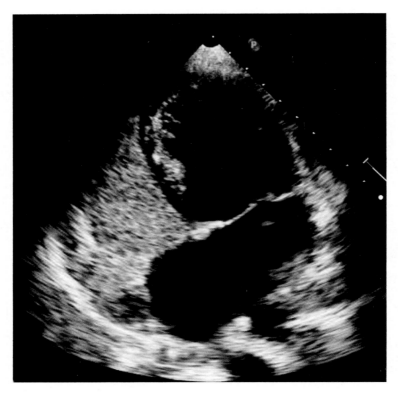

FIGURE 24-8. Atrial septal aneurysm.

Congenital Heart Disorders

CHAPTER 25

GUIDELINES

Baumgartner H, Bonhoeffer P, De Groot NM, et al. ESC Guidelines for the management of grown-up congenital heart disease. Eur Heart J. 2010;31:2915–2957.

Comprehensive reference from Europe.

Stout KK, Daniels CJ, Aboulhosn JA, et al. 2018 AHA/ACC Guideline for the **Management** of Adults With Congenital Heart Disease. Circulation. 2019;139:e698–e800.

Find the disorder in the table of contents. Read the synopsis.

Warnes CA, Williams RG, Bashore TM, et al. ACC/AHA 2008 Guidelines for the Management of Adults with Congenital Heart Disease. Circulation. 2008;118:e714–e833.

Authoritative comprehensive reference. Written by experts in the field.

Echo Imaging References

Khraiche D, Ben Moussa N. Assessment of right ventricular systolic function by echocardiography **after surgical repair** of congenital heart defects. Arch Cardiovasc Dis. 2016;109:113–119.

Postoperative impairment of RV systolic function can appear after surgical repair of complex congenital heart defects, such as tetralogy of Fallot. It is caused by chronic volume and/or pressure overload due to pulmonary regurgitation and/or stenosis. RV dysfunction is strongly associated with prognosis in these patients.

Simpson J, Lopez L, Acar P, et al. **Three-dimensional** echocardiography in congenital heart disease. Eur Heart J Cardiovasc Imaging. 2016;17:1071–1097.

Sreedhar R. Acyanotic congenital heart disease and transesophageal echocardiography. Ann Card Anaesth. 2017;20(Supplement):S36–S42.

TEE findings in congenital heart defects.

Vettukattil JJ. Three-dimensional echocardiography in congenital heart disease. Heart. 2012;98:79–88.

Follow this author if you are interested in 3D printing of congenital heart defects.

See also: 3dprint.nih.gov/collections/heart-library.

ATRIAL SEPTAL DEFECT

Embryology

- It is important to understand the embryologic formation of the atrial septum.
- There is a complex septation process that includes sequential tissue connections, as well as tissue reabsorption by programmed cell death.
- The secundum atrial septal defect is actually a defect of the primum septum.
- The primum septum grows to divide the originally single embryologic atrium into two atria.
- At the same time, the endocardial cushions are growing to separate the atria from the ventricles.
- The septum primum grows toward the endocardial cushions.
- As the primum septum grows, fenestrations develop, creating the ostium secundum.
- Tip: Easiest way to learn this is to watch a YouTube video on the embryology of the atrial septum.

Anderson RH, Brown NA, Webb S. **Development** and structure of the atrial septum. Heart. 2002;88:104–110.

Campbell M. **Natural history** of atrial septal defect. Br Heart J. 1970;32:820–826.

Craig RJ, Selzer A. Natural history and **prognosis** of atrial septal defect. Circulation. 1968;37:805–815.

Saxena A, Divekar A, Soni NR. Natural history of secundum atrial septal defect revisited in the era of **transcatheter closure**. Indian Heart J. 2005;57:35–38.

Webb G, Gatzoulis MA. Atrial septal defects in the adult: recent progress and **overview**. Circulation. 2006;114:1645–1653.

Secundum Atrial Septal Defect

- A secundum atrial septal defect may be diagnosed for the first time in an adult patient.
- The patient may be referred for an echo because of fixed splitting of the second heart sound on auscultation.
- The patient may relate that a lifelong systolic murmur at the upper left sternal border had been repeatedly dismissed in the past as an innocent flow murmur.
- Cardiac catheterization is rarely performed nowadays to calculate the size of the shunt by measuring the increased oxygen saturation in the right atrium.
- A secundum ASD is a defect in the central portion of the atrial septum (Fig. 25-1).
- It has been referred to as the only true defect of the atrial septum—all other defects being more complicated in nature (see the subsequent discussions in this chapter). It is also the only defect at this time that can be treated by percutaneous device closure.
- Scanning tips:
  - A transthoracic echo in an adult may *not* make the diagnosis of an ASD conclusively.
  - It is important to look at the pulmonic valve morphology carefully at the time the diagnosis of a secundum ASD is made, or suspected.
  - Valvular pulmonic stenosis is associated with secundum ASD.
  - The increased ASD shunt flow velocities across the pulmonic valve may be mistaken for pulmonic stenosis.

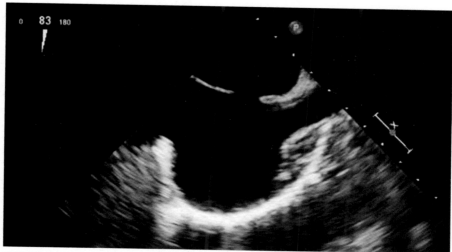

FIGURE 25-1. Secundum atrial septal defect.

- TEE is performed in the adult secundum ASD patient to:
  - Confirm the diagnosis.
  - Obtain better detail of the atrial septal defect size, 3D contour, and rim tissue.
  - Look for other abnormalities, such as anomalous pulmonary veins.
  - Help in planning the treatment: The tissue rim around the defect can be measured for feasibility of percutaneous device closure.
- Ideally, at least 5 mm of rim tissue is needed to securely deploy a closure device.

ECHO DROPOUT OF THE FOSSA OVALIS MEMBRANE

- The best 2D images are obtained when ultrasound strikes tissue at a perpendicular 90 degrees.
- Unfortunately, in the apical views, the thin fossa ovalis membrane is positioned parallel to the ultrasound beam.
- It is therefore *perfectly normal* for an echo dropout to be present at the atrial septum in the apical four-chamber view.
- To the untrained observer who has not read this book, this normal echocardiographic appearance may wrongly suggest the presence of a secundum atrial septal defect.

SINUS VENOSUS ATRIAL SEPTAL DEFECT

"Dilated RV—Think SV ASD—Do a TEE"

- This is a defect of the infolding of the atrial roof where it normally separates the superior vena cava from the right upper pulmonary vein.
- It can be diagnosed only when the rim of the fossa ovalis is present.
- The defect overrides the rim.

- The superior vena cava overrides the defect and has a biatrial connection.
- It is interatrial but is considered extracardiac from an embryologic perspective.
- It is frequently missed on transthoracic echo in the adult.
- The right atrium and right ventricle are dilated.
- TEE is usually necessary in the adult to identify the abnormal right pulmonary venous drainage, and to demonstrate the defect.

al Zaghal AM, Li J, Anderson RH, et al. **Anatomical criteria** for the diagnosis of sinus venosus defects. Heart. 1997;78: 298–304.

Van Praagh S, Carrera ME, Sanders SP, et al. Sinus venosus defects: unroofing of the right pulmonary veins—anatomic and echocardiographic findings and surgical treatment. Am Heart J. 1994;128:365–379.

DILATED CORONARY SINUS

- The presence of a dilated coronary sinus in PLAX should prompt a search for a persistent left superior vena cava.
- Pitfall: When scanning a significantly dilated coronary sinus from the apical position, an inexperienced interpreter may mistake the abnormal anatomic appearance for a primum atrial septal defect.

PERSISTENT LEFT SUPERIOR VENA CAVA (PLSVC)

"Scrutinize the size of the coronary sinus in the first few seconds of looking at every PLAX image."

- Suspect PLSVC if the coronary sinus is dilated.
- An injection of agitated saline in a left arm vein will go from the left superior vena cava, to the coronary sinus, to the *right* atrium.
- There are misconceptions when it comes to a superior vena cava on the left side of the chest.
  - This is simply an extra systemic vein.
  - PLSVC is *not* a pulmonary vein.
  - There is no arteriovenous shunt unless there is unroofing of the coronary sinus (see below).
  - PLSVC alone does not require intervention.
- A dilated coronary sinus in PLAX may be mistaken for:
  - Descending thoracic aortic aorta.
  - Localized pericardial effusion.
  - Pericardial cyst.
- Pacemakers and PLSVC:
  - Pacemakers are routinely implanted on the *left* side of the chest.
  - Problems are caused by someone unaware of the anatomy, advancing a catheter or a wire into the PLSVC tract continuous with the coronary sinus.
  - This can cause arrhythmias, hemodynamic instability, or perforation of the heart.

- Cardioplegia and PLSVC:
  - In patients undergoing cardioplegia for open heart surgery, it is important to diagnose PLSVC because the cardioplegia will become ineffective and therefore potentially dangerous for the patient.
  - PLSVC results in excessive runoff of cardioplegia solution into the persistent left superior vena cava, and into the right atrium.
  - It is possible to technically modify the procedure, and it has been possible to perform cardioplegia in patients with PLSVC.

Biffi M, Boriani G, Frabetti L, et al. Left superior vena cava persistence in patients undergoing pacemaker or cardioverter-defibrillator implantation: a 10-year experience. Chest. 2001;120:139–144.

Fernando RJ, Johnson SD. Inability to utilize retrograde cardioplegia due to a persistent left superior vena cava. Case Rep Anesthesiol. 2017;4671856.

CORONARY SINUS ATRIAL SEPTAL DEFECT

- This defect is not located in the atrial septum.
- Unroofing of the coronary sinus as it travels behind the left atrium allows communication from the left atrium to the right atrium via the unroofed coronary sinus.
- A persistent left superior vena cava is commonly associated with this defect.
- Parasternal long-axis images will demonstrate a dilated coronary sinus.
- Color flow may show the unroofing and communication to the left atrium.
- An injection of agitated saline in a left arm vein will go from the coronary sinus to the *left* atrium, and to the *left* ventricle.
- The clinical presentation is similar to that of an atrial septal defect, with the addition of transient exertional cyanosis in some patients.

*Chen C, Xu L, Xu Y, et al. Unroofed coronary sinus syndrome: an easily corrected congenital anomaly but more **diagnostic suspicion** is needed. Heart Lung Circ. 2018;27:731–738.*

VENTRICULAR SEPTAL DEFECT

- The ventricular septum has four embryologic components.
- Failure in the development of a component is responsible for the corresponding type of ventricular septal defect.
  1. Invagination of embryologic myocardium forms the *muscular* ventricular septum.
     - A small muscular ventricular septal defect may close spontaneously over time. There is usually a rim of muscle around the defect. The mitral and tricuspid valves are not affected by the defect.
     - *Acquired* muscular ventricular septal defects are a highly lethal complication of myocardial infarction.
  2. The *inlet* ventricular septum is formed by the endocardial cushions that are growing in the fetus to separate the atria from the ventricles.
     - Patients with Down syndrome have a high incidence of inlet AV canal defects of the endocardial cushions.
     - The AV valves are abnormal, and surgical repair may be required.

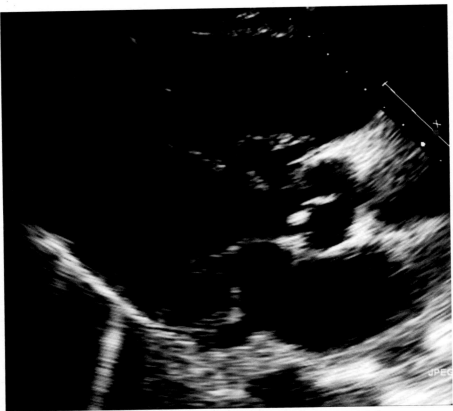

FIGURE 25-2. Aneurysmal transformation of a healed ventricular septal defect.

3. The outlet region of the ventricular septum is the *conotruncal* septum.

   - Tetralogy of Fallot is a complex conotruncal abnormality that includes a ventricular septal defect.
   - Supracristal ventricular septal defects are located past the crista supraventricularis of the right ventricular outflow. This defect results in lack of muscular support for the nearby right aortic valve cusp.

4. The connection of the aorta to the ventricular septum can be incomplete.

   - A *membranous* (also called perimembranous) ventricular septal defect is located in the thinnest part of the septum, at the base. It is located between the aortic and tricuspid valves. It can be spontaneously closed over time by overgrowth of tricuspid valve tissue. This is called *aneurysmal transformation* (Fig. 25-2).

Enseleit F, Reho I, Largiadèr T, et al. Continuous wave Doppler signal: a mystery. J Am Soc Echocardiogr. 2006;19:1191.

Fraisse A, Massih TA, Bonnet D, et al. Cleft of the mitral valve in patients with **Down's** syndrome. Cardiol Young. 2002;12:27–31.

Mitral regurgitation in a patient with Down syndrome should prompt 3D examination of the valve.

Fraisse A, Massih TA, Kreitmann B, et al. Characteristics and management of **cleft mitral** valve. J Am Coll Cardiol. 2003;42:1988–1993.

A cleft can be present with or without an AV canal defect.

Scanning Technique for Ventricular Septal Defects

- Begin with 2D imaging of the smooth left ventricular surface of the interventricular septum.
- Learn to follow the contour and complex curvature of the septum with 2D.
- It is usually more difficult to find the defect with 2D on the trabeculated irregular right ventricular septum. Stick to the left side of the septum with your 2D sweeps.
- Practice performing a slow apex-to-base 2D sweep in the parasternal window. Look for an echo dropout on the left ventricular endocardial surface.
- Perform a slow 2D apical window sweep of the ventricular septum that starts at the "floor" where you see the coronary sinus; continue to tilt the transducer anteriorly, following the left ventricular border of the interventricular septum until you get to the aorta in the "five-chamber" view.
- Color flow and pulsed-wave Doppler in the right ventricle will confirm the 2D finding.
- There may be a PISA on the left ventricular side of the defect.

Hemodynamic Importance

- The hemodynamic impact of a ventricular septal defect depends on the size.
- For example, a small restrictive ventricular septal defect is suspected from a loud systolic murmur. The patient is asymptomatic. Echo is performed to confirm the diagnosis, but no treatment is needed.
- At the other extreme, a large unrepaired ventricular septal defect with an unobstructed path to the lungs can lead to lethal, irreversible pulmonary hypertension.

QP:QS BASICS

In the absence of shunts, QP = QS.

Pulmonary flow examples:
QP: Flow arriving at the lungs via the pulmonary artery.
QP: Flow arriving in the left atrium from the pulmonary veins.

Systemic flow examples:
QS: Flow going to the body via the aorta.
QS: Flow arriving at the right atrium from the superior and inferior vena cava.
- Shunt calculations are done by calculating stroke volume at different valves and comparing it.
- In the absence of shunts (or valve regurgitation), the calculated stroke volume should be the same at each valve.
- This "ratio of blue blood to red blood" can be calculated in ASD, VSD, and PDA.

Sanders SP, Yeager S, Williams RG. Measurement of systemic and pulmonary blood flow and QP/QS ratio using Doppler and two-dimensional echocardiography. Am J Cardiol. 1983;51:952–956.

- Two scanning tips with suspected ventricular septal defects:
  1. Transthoracic echo in the cath lab.
     - The package inserts of echocardiographic contrast agents warn not to administer to patients with known or suspected right-to-left, bidirectional, or transient right-to-left shunts, and not to administer by intra-arterial injection.
     - On the other hand, imaging with ultrasound during a standard *radiologic contrast* left ventriculogram performed in the catheterization laboratory may help in the echocardiographic localization of the left-to-right shunt of a suspected ventricular septal defect.
  2. Doppler jet direction.

     In the parasternal short axis views, a restrictive ventricular septal defect is diagnosed as a high-velocity systolic jet coming *toward* the transducer.
     - In the apical views, a rare patient with severe aortic stenosis may show a pericardial mirror reflection of the aortic stenosis jet *back toward* the transducer. This may be mistaken for a jet from an undiagnosed ventricular septal defect.
     - To determine the origin of an unknown Doppler signal, it may be useful to geometrically reconstruct the pathway of the ultrasound beam as described by Enseleit et al.

Note: Multiple imaging windows should always be used in the Doppler evaluation of aortic stenosis.

Enseleit F, Reho I, Largiadèr T, et al. Continuous wave Doppler signal: a mystery. J Am Soc Echocardiogr. 2006;19:1191.

DOUBLE-CHAMBERED RIGHT VENTRICLE

- A ventricular septal defect color flow jet can sometimes enter a double-chambered right ventricle.
- There are hypertrophic muscle bands dividing this right ventricle into a high-pressure proximal inlet chamber.
- There is a distal, low-pressure outlet right ventricular chamber located downstream from the obstruction.
- Echo can demonstrate:
  - The gradient and direction of flow across the ventricular septal defect.
  - The gradient across the muscle bands in the right ventricle. This gradient can increase over time.
- Note: The muscle bands that divide the right ventricle may be better visualized from the subcostal window.
  - It can localize the entry point of the VSD to the inlet or outlet chamber.
- Caution: A high tricuspid regurgitation velocity from the proximal high-pressure inlet chamber may falsely suggest the presence of pulmonary hypertension.

Lascano ME, Schaad MS, Moodie DS, et al. Difficulty in diagnosing double-chambered right ventricle in adults. Am J Cardiol. 2001;88:816–819.

EMBRYOLOGY OF L-TRANSPOSITION

- Normal cardiac development:
  - During normal cardiac development, the embryologic cardiac tube is eventually transformed into a four-chambered heart.
  - In order for this to happen, there is folding of the growing cardiac tube because it is constrained by the slower growing pericardium. (Think of soft-serve ice cream being crammed into a constraining ice cream cone.)
  - The folding process of the embryologic cardiac tube is called *looping*.
  - Normal looping is convex and to the right: D-looping.
  - Normal D-looping results in the right ventricle being anterior and to the right, and the left ventricle being positioned posterior and to the left.
  - Connection to the great vessels: The embryologic tubelike trunk of the aorta and pulmonary artery grows in spiral fashion.
  - As the great vessels grow and separate normally, the normal origin of the aorta is posterior and to the left—normally connecting to the left ventricle. The normal origin of the pulmonary artery is anterior and to the right—connecting to the normal right ventricle.
- L-transposition:
  - If the cardiac loop twists to the left instead of to the right, the right ventricle becomes positioned posteriorly and to the left. If it connects to the aorta from this position, it can become the systemic ventricle.

ECHO IMAGING OF TRANSPOSITION

"With unoperated D-TGA you D-ie."

"With L-TGA you L-ive."

- The following are some useful echo imaging tips and concepts when evaluating adult patients with a diagnosis of "transposition."
- It is advisable to refrain from saying "left ventricle" and "right ventricle."
- The terms *venous ventricle* and *systemic ventricle* are less confusing.
- Agitated saline contrast can help identify the venous chambers.
- The fortuitous presence of a pacemaker wire identifies that ventricle as venous. The other ventricle can then be called systemic.
- If it is possible to demonstrate a bifurcation in a great vessel, it can be used to identify it as the pulmonary artery.
- The native semilunar valve goes with its corresponding great vessel. The pulmonic valve goes with the vessel that branches (pulmonary artery). The aortic valve goes with the vessel that arches (aorta).
- Once the pulmonary artery has been identified, the semilunar valve in the pulmonary artery is the pulmonic valve.
- Coronary ostia in a great vessel identify it as the aorta, and the native semilunar valve in the aorta is the aortic valve. (Exception to this rule: See ALCAPA)

- In the subcostal view, it is important to identify the suprahepatic segment of the inferior vena cava, which always drains into the right atrium. This helps to identify the atria as right and left.
- The native atrioventricular valve goes with its corresponding ventricle: The mitral valve goes with the left ventricle. The tricuspid valve goes with the right ventricle.
- If an atrioventricular valve is shown on echo to be in direct contact with a semilunar valve, the two valves are said to be in *fibrous continuity*.
- A ventricle with an infundibulum can be called the anatomic right ventricle.
- A ventricle that has atrioventricular and semilunar valves in fibrous continuity has no infundibulum to separate them, and it can be postulated to be the anatomic left ventricle.
- Once the atria, ventricles, and great vessels are identified, echo imaging can proceed to demonstrate the connections.

Cohen MS, Eidem BW, Cetta F, et al. Multimodality **imaging guidelines** of patients with transposition of the great arteries. J Am Soc Echocardiogr. 2016;29:571–621.

Hornung TS, Calder L. **Congenitally corrected** transposition of the great arteries. Heart. 2010;96:1154–1161.

There is usually normal drainage of the systemic and pulmonary veins to the right and left atria respectively.

The right atrium connects via the mitral valve to the morphologic left ventricle, which supplies the pulmonary artery.

The left atrium connects via the tricuspid valve to the morphologic right ventricle, which supplies the aorta via a subaortic infundibulum.

The ventricles are most commonly side by side: In patients with situs solitus the morphologic left ventricle is rightward and the morphologic right ventricle is leftward.

Warnes CA. Transposition of the great arteries. Circulation. 2006;114:2699–2709.

Comprehensive review article.

THE THEBESIAN VALVE OF THE CORONARY SINUS

- Small fold of endocardium at the opening of the coronary sinus.
- It is only occasionally visible on echo imaging.
- It may obstruct variable amounts of the coronary sinus opening.
- It may be fenestrated and may obstruct retrograde entry of a pacemaker wire or cardioplegia catheter.

Kuroda M, Takahashi T, Mita N, et al. Difficult cannulation of the coronary sinus due to a large Thebesian valve. Anesth Analg. 2013;116:563–566.

Vander Salm TJ. Coronary sinus cannulation: a technique to overcome an obstructing Thebesian valve. Ann Thorac Surg. 1993;56:1441–1442.

CHAPTER 26

The Stethoscope

COLOR FLOW DOPPLER AND HEART MURMURS

- The finding of mitral or aortic regurgitation on color flow should prompt a search for the corresponding murmur.
- An absent murmur when there is evidence of severe regurgitation on color flow needs an explanation.
- The echocardiographic explanation of a murmur may reside in the left ventricle: hypertrophy, outflow obstruction, chamber dilatation, mitral annulus dilatation.
- Color flow Doppler is highly capable of detecting valvular regurgitation.
- It is an instantaneous spatial display of mean blood flow velocities—different from an angiogram.
- Regurgitant murmurs are commonly found by color flow Doppler without being heard on auscultation.
- Connecting color flow with a murmur is not always straightforward, but correlation of the color flow Doppler exam with auscultation is extremely valuable clinically.
- Innocent flow murmurs may become audible in the recumbent position due to increased venous return. There is no color flow Doppler equivalent to a murmur caused by normal forward flow through the right cardiac chambers.
- Turbulent blood flow is displayed with a variance map on color flow, and by spectral broadening on pulsed-wave Doppler.
- Practical example: A sclerotic aortic valve may give rise to a prominent systolic ejection murmur, but there will be no significant gradient on pulsed- and continuous-wave Doppler.
- Color flow Doppler is useful during the assessment of the severity of aortic stenosis. Multiple transducer positions are used to align the continuous-wave Doppler beam with the stenotic jet. Color flow can help find the turbulent flow in the aorta in the right parasternal and suprasternal transducer positions during the "hunt" for the fastest aortic stenosis velocity.

- Bedside scanning tip: Palpate for the thrill of the aortic stenosis murmur first, and place the transducer directly over that spot on the chest.

Yoshida K, Yoshikawa J, Shakudo M, et al. Color Doppler evaluation of valvular regurgitation in normal subjects. Circulation. 1988;78:840–847.

SYSTOLIC EJECTION MURMURS

- The Doppler flow pattern can help sort out a systolic ejection murmur by providing the following parameters:
  - Time of systolic peaking.
  - Onset in relation to the isovolumic period.
  - Ejection time.
- The peak of a systolic Doppler flow signal through the aortic valve can be correlated with the auscultatory impression of whether an aortic murmur peaks early or late in systole.
- Systolic ejection murmurs *end before* the second heart sound.
- There is an auscultation "caveat" that may help the listener decide whether the murmur stops before the second heart sound (making it an ejection-type murmur).
- This only works with loud murmurs where it is clear to the listener that the murmur is louder than the second heart sound.
- The caveat goes as follows: If the listener hears a second heart sound that is softer than the preceding systolic murmur, it means that the murmur *stops* before the second heart sound.
- This auscultatory impression can be confirmed by the Doppler flow pattern.
- Pulsed-wave Doppler can show the *turbulence* of a murmur by exhibiting spectral broadening.

THE SECOND HEART SOUND IN AORTIC STENOSIS

- Over time, in worsening aortic stenosis, the aortic component of the second heart sound (A2) progressively decreases in intensity.
- It tends to disappear completely in severe aortic stenosis.
- The pulmonic component of the second heart sound remains audible.
- How to determine at the bedside that A2 is decreased or absent:
  - The bedside exam should start with identification of the heart sounds. Murmurs should initially be ignored.
  - One must compare the second heart sound at the *left* upper sternal border to the second heart sound in the *right* upper sternal border.
  - In the absence of pulmonary hypertension, the pulmonic component of the second heart sound is confined to the upper *left* sternal border.

- At the upper *right* sternal border the second heart sound should not have components from the pulmonic valve, and it should therefore be influenced only by the degree of aortic valve mobility.

Chandraratna PA, Lopez JM, Cohen LS. Echocardiographic observations on the mechanism of production of the second heart sound. Circulation. 1975;51:292–296.

S2 is caused by deceleration of columns of blood resulting from semilunar valve closure.

MURMUR OF AORTIC STENOSIS

- The murmur of aortic stenosis is typically loud enough *not* to be missed on physical examination.
- It is best heard at the upper right sternal border and transmits to the neck.
- Loudness does *not* correlate with severity.
- The murmur has a crescendo–decrescendo ejection quality that can be confirmed with Doppler.
- In order to estimate the severity of aortic stenosis on auscultation, one must train the ear to recognize a murmur that is *peaking late* as opposed to a non-obstructive ejection murmur that peaks in early to mid systole.
- The best way to hone this bedside skill is by feedback. The *contour* of the aortic stenosis Doppler signal correlates with the peaking of the murmur. It can be used as feedback to refine the auscultatory impression.

GALLAVARDIN PHENOMENON

- The Gallavardin phenomenon is diagnosed by using color flow Doppler in conjunction with auscultation.
- It refers to an *auscultatory dissociation* of the aortic stenosis murmur in some patients. The same murmur sounds remarkably different at the apex and at the base.
- The aortic stenosis murmur in these patients is harsh and noisy (as usual) at the base, but paradoxically soft, blowing, and musical at the apex.
- Although any experienced clinician knows that mitral regurgitation is frequently associated with aortic stenosis, the auscultatory impression of *combined* aortic stenosis and mitral regurgitation may be wrong in patients with the Gallavardin phenomenon.
- Absence of mitral regurgitation on color flow Doppler confirms the presence of the Gallavardin phenomenon in aortic stenosis patients with a musical apical "mitral" murmur.

Gallavardin L. Pauper-Ravault. Le souffle' du retrecissement aortique puet changer de timbre et devenir dans sa propagation apexienne. Lyon Med. 1925:523.

Giles TD, Martinez EC, Burch GE. Gallavardin phenomenon in aortic stenosis. A possible mechanism. Arch Intern Med. 1974;134:747–749.

MURMUR IN THE BACK

- The following echocardiographic findings help sort out the cause for a murmur heard in the back:
  - Mitral valve prolapse.
  - Hypertrophic cardiomyopathy.
  - Bicuspid aortic valve.
  - Pulmonic stenosis.
- The mitral regurgitation jet of *anterior* mitral valve prolapse is directed "opposite the culprit leaflet." It is therefore directed posteriorly and may be heard in the back, in the interscapular region.
- Systolic anterior motion of the mitral valve in hypertrophic cardiomyopathy may direct the mitral regurgitation jet to the posterior left atrial wall.
- Bicuspid aortic valve is associated with coarctation of the aorta. The murmur of coarctation is heard in the back.
- The jet of valvular pulmonic stenosis favors the left main branch of the pulmonary artery. The murmur is widely disseminated across the chest and is also directed to the back.

HEART SOUNDS IN ATRIAL FIBRILLATION

- Variable intensity of heart sounds is a known auscultatory finding in atrial fibrillation.
- There are echocardiographic equivalents:
  - M-mode of aortic valve opening shows beat-to-beat variability of aortic leaflet opening.
  - There is beat-to-beat variability in stroke volume VTI.

Abelson D. Ultrasonic Doppler auscultation of the heart, with observations on atrial flutter and fibrillation. JAMA. 1968; 204:438–443.

THE AORTIC EJECTION CLICK

- A loud first heart sound at the upper right sternal border may be a manifestation of an ejection click that cannot be separated from the first heart sound by the listener—making it perceptibly louder.
- The findings to note on echo are:
  - Doming of aortic leaflets in a bicuspid valve.
  - Dilatation of the aorta.

EJECTION CLICK VERSUS ATRIAL GALLOP

- The auscultatory hallmark of a bicuspid aortic valve is the early systolic ejection click.
- This ejection click must be distinguished at the bedside from a normally split first heart sound, and from an atrial gallop (S4).

- The ejection click is a short, sharp sound that is easily heard both at the aortic area on the right side of the sternum, and equally well (or better) at the apex.
- The normal first heart sound never splits at the upper right sternal border (only at the lower left sternal border where the tricuspid component is normally present).
- Normal splitting of the first heart sound is typically heard in a limited area at the lower left sternal border where the tricuspid closure component (T1) is heard— contributing to the splitting of M1 (mitral closure component) and T1.
- A left atrial gallop is heard only at the apex. It is usually a difficult-to-hear low-frequency "thud." The bell of the stethoscope is pressed lightly against the skin with just enough pressure to create a seal and eliminate entry of distracting ambient noise via the bell. Further pressure may actually *filter out* the gallop by stretching the skin and "creating a diaphragm." Varying the pressure of the bell to intermittently muffle the gallop during auscultation can be used to confirm its presence by making it "come and go" (Fig. 26-1).
- Caution: Patients with right bundle branch block on the electrocardiogram frequently have a widely split first heart sound at the left lower sternal border. This may get confused with an atrial gallop. Look at the ECG before you open your mouth.

Vancheri F, Gibson D. Relation of third and fourth heart sounds to blood velocity during left ventricular filling. Br Heart J. 1989;61:144–148.

PULMONIC EJECTION CLICK

- Patients with pulmonic valve stenosis have a unique, potentially diagnostic finding on auscultation.

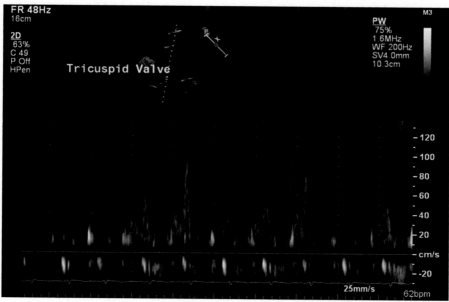

FIGURE 26-1. Respiratory variation identifies S4 gallops as right sided.

- There is an early systolic ejection click with unique behavior. The click gets louder on *expiration*.
- There is no accepted echocardiographic equivalent.
- However, the M-mode of the pulmonic valve has its own unique behavior in pulmonic stenosis: It opens a crack with the atrial contraction and remains open until the end of systole.

VENTRICULAR S3 GALLOP

- Just like the restrictive mitral inflow pattern on pulsed-wave Doppler, an S3 gallop is normal in healthy young patients but ominous in adults (and in children) with heart failure.

ATRIAL S4 GALLOP

- There are multiple echocardiographic equivalents for the S4 gallop. It remains an important marker of diastolic dysfunction (Fig. 26-2).

Tavel ME. Editorial: The fourth heart sound—a premature requiem? Circulation. 1974;49:4–6.

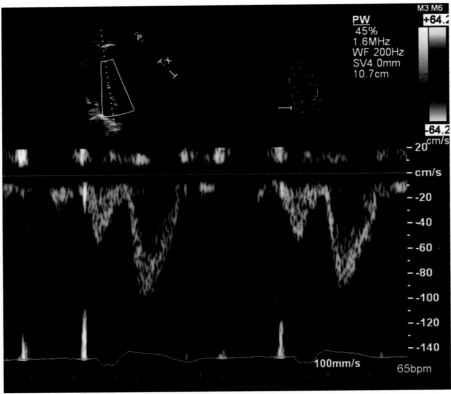

FIGURE 26-2. Pulsed-wave Doppler "equivalent" of the S4 gallop.

THE SECOND HEART SOUND

- When there is a right bundle branch block on the ECG, the normal inspiratory splitting of the second heart sound becomes *exaggerated* and easier to hear.
- Patients with right ventricular pacemakers and with left bundle branch block on the ECG have an abnormally split second heart sound. This is called *paradoxical* splitting: The second heart sound splits in expiration and becomes single on inspiration.
- By regularly listening to those patients with your stethoscope, you will hone your auscultation skills. Pay attention to the splitting behavior of the second heart sound while the patient continues to breathe normally.
- *Fixed* splitting of the second heart sound is an important clue to the presence of an atrial septal defect.

Luisada AA. *The second heart sound in normal and abnormal conditions. Am J Cardiol. 1971;28:150–161.*

Shindler DM. *Effect of the Valsalva maneuver on the second heart sound. Cardiology. 2018;139:159–160.*

THE FIRST HEART SOUND

- The tissue Doppler isovolumic velocities coincide in time with the multiple components of the first heart sound (S1).
- The loudness of the first heart sound is increased in mitral stenosis.
- A short PR on ECG, or a hyperdynamic cardiac state (tachycardia, hyperthyroidism), also will *increase* S1 loudness.
- A long PR on ECG will *decrease* S1 loudness.
- Both mitral and tricuspid regurgitation start during the isovolumic period— *decreasing* the loudness of the mitral and tricuspid components of S1, respectively.

MITRAL STENOSIS OPENING SNAP

- This is an early diastolic sound that is heard at the time of the Doppler E wave in mitral stenosis.
- Hearing an opening snap should prompt the performance of an echo for confirmation of the diagnosis of mitral stenosis.

AUSCULTATION OF AN OPENING SNAP

"Echocardiography can be useful for determining the reason why the opening snap is conspicuously difficult to hear in some known mitral stenosis patients."

- The loud first heart sound of mitral stenosis, followed by the second heart sound (made louder if there is pulmonary hypertension), and followed by the (usually) loud opening snap, combine to give *an unmistakable* loud *triple rhythm* on auscultation.
- A heavily calcified, immobile stenotic mitral valve (easily shown on echo) is no longer pliable, and both the loud first heart sound and the loud opening snap

decrease in intensity, or actually become inaudible on auscultation. Moderate to severe mitral regurgitation (perhaps due to prior mitral valvuloplasty) may mask or attenuate the *first* heart sound.

- The opening snap may come earlier because of elevated left atrial pressure and may "blend in" with the *second* heart sound on auscultation.
- The opening snap may be *misinterpreted* on auscultation as a widely split second heart sound (if the diagnosis of mitral stenosis is not suspected, or echo is not available).
- But if there is *no* bundle branch block on the ECG, why should the "second heart sound" be so widely split?
- Raising the legs during auscultation (to increase venous return) may help sort this out: The second heart sound splits *more* with *increased* venous return, because pulmonic valve closure gets delayed.
- The interval between an audibly single second heart sound and the opening snap does the opposite when the legs are raised.
- Increased venous return elevates left atrial pressure, and the mitral valve "snaps open" earlier, hence closer to the second heart sound.
- It may also help to pay attention to the respiratory cycle. A widely split second heart sound may still perceptibly change with respiration.

THE DIASTOLIC RUMBLE OF MITRAL STENOSIS

- The diastolic rumble of mitral stenosis is notoriously difficult to hear and to recognize on auscultation.
- The bell of the stethoscope is held lightly at the point of apical impulse with just enough pressure on the skin to create a seal that blocks out ambient noise.
- The low-frequency nature of this diastolic flow murmur through the stenotic mitral valve orifice has been compared to "distant thunder," or to a "rolling bowling ball."
- There is a presystolic accentuation in the rumble, caused by atrial contraction. The presystolic component of the diastolic rumble "fluffs out" the first heart sound by blending into it.
- The unique combination of acoustic phenomena in mitral stenosis allows an experienced examiner to *make the diagnosis* of mitral stenosis on auscultation.

VENOUS HUM

"Normal echo in a patient referred for a continuous murmur."

- A continuous murmur is usually considered to be evidence of a patent ductus arteriosus, but patent ductus arteriosus is *rare* after the neonatal period.
- On physical examination of a young patient (usually in their early teens) it is quite *common* to discover the presence of an innocent continuous murmur—the venous hum.
- When recognized as such by the examiner, a venous hum does not require a referral for an echocardiogram.

- Auscultatory features:
  - The venous hum is heard during auscultation of the right side of the neck in the *sitting* position.
  - It is due to torrential venous flow from the head vessels to the right heart in young patients with very compliant right cardiac chambers. It is (to put it simply) driven by gravity. It disappears in the recumbent position.
  - The loudness of this murmur increases on the right side of the neck when the patient's head is turned to the left (because the caliber of the right jugular vein is narrowed and blood flow becomes even more turbulent).
  - This innocent continuous murmur may, in some cases, transmit and extend to the chest—making it prone to misinterpretation. When this innocent murmur is heard in the chest, the first inclination may be to diagnose a patent ductus arteriosus.
  - The "cure" for this presumed patent ductus arteriosus is very simple. Compressing the neck with the examiner's finger just *above* the stethoscope will make the murmur completely disappear (by stopping blood flow).
  - The prominent bounding arterial pulse of patent ductus arteriosus is "conspicuous by being absent" in the patient with an innocent venous hum.
  - The only other consideration is that a venous hum and a patent ductus arteriosus are not mutually exclusive, and *both* may be present in the same patient. If the continuous murmur continues to be heard in the recumbent position, an echocardiogram *is* indicated.

AUSCULTATION IN PATENT DUCTUS ARTERIOSUS

- The murmur of a persistently patent ductus in an adult may sometimes only be systolic rather than the typical continuous "machinery" murmur.
- The typical murmur increases in intensity throughout systole, becoming loudest at the time of aortic valve closure. It *continues* without interruption into diastole, decreasing in intensity but assuming a higher frequency.
  - There may be "shaking dice" noises, or multiple clicks in systole.
  - Increased flow through the mitral valve may result in an apical diastolic rumble.
- The ductus murmur is distinguished from a venous hum by the location where it is heard loudest and by turning the head during auscultation.
- The hum changes when the head is turned.
- Hums are modified by respiration, and by a change in body position.
- The ductal murmur is loudest at the second left intercostal space.
- The venous hum may be loudest at the supraclavicular fossa, or on the right side of the sternum.
- Other causes of continuous murmurs:
  - Ruptured sinus of Valsalva aneurysm.
  - Coronary artery fistula.
  - Aortopulmonary window.
  - Collateral flow murmurs in tetralogy of Fallot with pulmonary atresia.

- Tetralogy of Fallot with pulmonary atresia should always be considered in a cyanotic neonate with continuous murmurs heard over the back.

Forsey JT, Elmasry OA, Martin RP. Patent arterial duct. Orphanet J Rare Dis. 2009;4:17.

PLAX COLOR FLOW IN CONTINUOUS MURMURS

- A continuous murmur on auscultation in a patient will invariably get evaluated with an echocardiogram.
- The *location* of continuous color flow in PLAX in a patient with a continuous murmur can be used for diagnosis of four disorders. Three are rare disorders, usually diagnosed at a pediatric age, and one cannot be missed in an adult echo lab. It is a surgically treatable life-threatening acquired disorder.
- Continuous color flow:
  1. Below the aortic cusp—combined systolic flow from a subaortic ventricular septal defect and diastolic flow from aortic regurgitation of an unsupported aortic cusp.
  2. Above the aortic cusp but below the sino-tubular junction—the rare life-threatening disorder that cannot be missed in adult echo lab: ruptured sinus of Valsalva.
  3. Above the sino-tubular junction and emptying into the pulmonary artery— aortopulmonary window.
  4. Above the sino-tubular junction and emptying into the left ventricle— aorticoventricular tunnel.

STILL'S INNOCENT CHILDHOOD MURMUR

- Adapted from Still's *original description*:
  - It is found in children between the ages of 2 and 6 years.
  - *Twanging* sound, somewhat musical, like a tense string.
  - The usual location is just below the level of the left nipple, halfway between the left margin of the sternum and the vertical left nipple line.
  - It is *not* heard in the axilla.
  - Audibility is variable during auscultation, being scarcely noticeable with some heart beats and being easily heard with others.
- Useful *observations by others*:
  - Low to medium pitch.
  - Early to mid systolic but separated from the first heart sound.
  - Loudness may vary from examination to examination.
  - It may be altered by respiration and by body position.
  - Lifting the legs in the recumbent position may make it louder. Try it while the patient is still in the lab if the echo is completely normal.
  - The murmur may be heard at the apex but is typically *not loudest* at the apex.
  - The quality of the murmur has been also described as *groaning, squeaking, croaking,* and *buzzing*.

Advani N, Menahem S, Wilkinson JL. The diagnosis of innocent murmurs in childhood. Cardiol Young. 2000;10:340–342.

CARDIOPULMONARY MURMUR

"An innocent murmur that will not be solved by performing an echocardiogram."

- Other names for the cardiopulmonary, or cardiorespiratory murmur:
  - Cardiopneumatic.
  - Extracardial.
  - Systolic vesicular.
- Description:
  - This is a superficial sounding murmur (seemingly heard "halfway up" the stethoscope).
  - There are flowery descriptions of the nature of the murmur.
  - It has been described as "bizarre," squealing, high pitched, blowing, and swishing, like the sound made by sipping hot soup, or like the puff of a steam locomotive.
  - It is most commonly found in young patients and may disappear as they get older.
  - As the multiple names imply, it may be heard at a border between the heart and the lungs.
  - The murmur is short and may start and stop abruptly.
  - It may disappear during different phases of respiration.
  - It may not coincide with a particular phase of the cardiac cycle.
  - It is usually localized, but the location where it is heard best varies from patient to patient.
  - It is said to be most commonly heard at the apex, but it can be localized to the left or right sternal borders or to the left infrascapular area in the back.
  - It will rarely transmit from where it is heard best—to the back, or to the axilla.

Practical example: A common circumstance where this murmur can come up for consideration is during daily routine cardiac auscultation. On first putting the stethoscope on the chest, it is not uncommon to form the auditory impression of a murmur. After a few respiratory cycles it becomes clear that the examiner is hearing *breath sounds*, and the "murmur" is dismissed by the examiner.

LOUD PULMONIC COMPONENT OF THE SECOND HEART SOUND

- The bedside diagnosis of a loud P2 requires practice and is best honed by correlating auscultatory and echocardiographic findings.
- The loudness of the second heart sound should be compared by listening at the upper left and at the upper right sternal border.
- The second heart sound can *split* at the upper left sternal border, but it should *not be louder* on the left.
- A split-second heart sound in pulmonary hypertension goes "up the musical scale."
- A loud P2 may radiate to the apex and to other areas of the chest. The listener should make sure there is no bundle branch block on the ECG to confound these findings.

AUSCULTATION OF PROSTHETIC VALVES

*Mitral versus aortic **mechanical** prosthesis.*

Mechanical valves may have a faint opening *click* on auscultation (in addition to the loud closure *click*). The challenge to the reader is to time the two different-sounding clicks along with the native closure sound and determine if the patient has a mitral or aortic mechanical prosthesis.

	S1	S2
Mitral mechanical on auscultation:	CLICK.........	Dub click
Aortic mechanical on auscultation:	Lub click......	CLICK
CLICK	= loud closure click	
Lub Dub	= native remaining valve closure sounds	
Faint click	= prosthesis opening ejection click	
....	= the dots represent systole	(S1[Lub]..........S2[Dub])

Echocardiography will easily determine mitral versus aortic location of a prosthesis, but it may sometimes come up short in distinguishing a mechanical from a biological prosthesis. In such cases, aside from asking the patient and using the stethoscope as discussed above, one can use fluoroscopy to image the prosthesis.

AUSCULTATION AND ECHOCARDIOGRAPHY DURING PREGNANCY

- Echocardiography is a safe and accepted tool for evaluation of cardiac disease during pregnancy.
- It is used in conjunction with the history, physical examination, and electrocardiogram.
- The cardiac evaluation seeks to determine the risk of continuing the pregnancy.
- Stenotic lesions increase risk, whereas regurgitant lesions typically do not.
- Marfan syndrome and severe pulmonary hypertension pose a prohibitive risk.
- Although a ventricular S3 gallop may be normal during late pregnancy, an atrial S4 gallop is not.
- Echo may be ordered during pregnancy for the following reasons:
  - New atrial S4 gallop.
  - New onset of hypertension.
  - Maternal congenital heart disease.
  - New arrhythmias.
  - New murmur.
  - New dyspnea on exertion.
- Progressive dyspnea on exertion is a common complaint in late pregnancy.
- Echocardiography plays a pivotal role in the evaluation of this typically benign, but potentially ominous symptom.
- Obstructive left heart lesions such as mitral stenosis should be suspected on the physical examination and should prompt an echocardiographic evaluation.
- Severe pulmonary hypertension is a *contraindication* to pregnancy.

- The decreased peripheral vascular resistance of pregnancy helps explain why atrial septal defects are usually well tolerated, and why the left-to-right shunt may not change for the worse as pregnancy progresses.
- The flow murmur of an undiagnosed atrial septal defect may get mistakenly *dismissed* on physical examination as an unusually loud flow murmur of pregnancy.

Penning S, Robinson KD, Major CA, et al. A comparison of echocardiography and pulmonary artery catheterization for evaluation of pulmonary artery pressures in pregnant patients with suspected pulmonary hypertension. Am J Obstet Gynecol. 2001;184:1568–1570.

Echocardiography overestimates pulmonary artery pressures compared with catheterization in pregnant patients.

Patients with structural cardiac defects appear to have a significantly greater discrepancy in pulmonary artery pressures.

One-third of pregnant patients with normal pulmonary artery pressures may be misclassified as having pulmonary artery hypertension.

Plethora of the inferior vena cava also is unreliable due to the volume overload of pregnancy.

Flow Murmur of Pregnancy

- The judicious use of echocardiography helps make the distinction between the common normal flow murmur of pregnancy and a pathologic murmur.
- Cardiac auscultation remains the diagnostic tool during routine follow-up visits.
- The nature of a flow murmur is different from that of a pathologic murmur:
  - Flow murmurs can change with body position and with respiration.
  - A flow murmur is usually *localized*—it is most likely to be heard at the upper left sternal border.
  - Loud systolic murmurs (and most diastolic murmurs) are likely to be pathologic rather than flow murmurs.

Mammary Souffle

"Continuous arterial murmur of pregnancy."
- It is due to enlarged tortuous branches of the internal mammary artery.
- It arises at the site of anastomosis between branches of aortic intercostal arteries and branches of the internal mammary artery, during the last month of pregnancy and during lactation.
- The murmur is obliterated by pressing down with the stethoscope, or by finger pressure next to the stethoscope.

Scott JT, Murphy EA. Mammary souffle of pregnancy: report of two cases simulating patent ductus arteriosus. Circulation. 1958;18:1038–1043.

Tabatznik B, Randall TW, Hersch C. The mammary souffle of pregnancy and lactation. Circulation. 1960;22:1069–1073.

NICOLADONI-BRANHAM SIGN

- Renal patients with arteriovenous fistulas may have unusually prominent Doppler color flow patterns in the right atrium due to increased venous return.

- This can be altered by using a large blood pressure cuff to occlude the fistula during echocardiographic imaging.
- During fistula occlusion, the color flow pattern will diminish. There should also be a reflex decrease in the heart rate (presumably due to decreased sympathetic tone).

Burchell HB. *Observations on bradycardia produced by occlusion of an artery proximal to an arteriovenous fistula (Nicoladoni-Branham sign). Med Clin North Am. 1958;42:1029–1035.*

Velez-Roa S, Neubauer J, Wissing M, et al. *Acute arteriovenous fistula occlusion decreases sympathetic activity and improves baroreflex control in kidney transplanted patients. Nephrol Dial Transplant. 2004;19:1606–1612.*

THE PERICARDIAL KNOCK IN CONSTRICTION

- The following bedside examination findings may be present in constriction:
  - Pericardial knock on auscultation.
  - Prominent jugular vein "y" descent.
  - Systolic retraction of the apical impulse.
  - Elevated venous pressure.
  - Kussmaul sign.
- Pericardial knock:
  - The pericardial knock can manifest as an unusually loud early diastolic third heart sound. It coincides with the mitral inflow E wave on echo.
  - It gets louder on squatting.
  - Even a relatively inexperienced clinician may recognize that there is a triple rhythm on auscultation.
  - Brief but brisk early diastolic right ventricular filling (that halts with the knock) causes the prominent "y" descent.
  - In constriction, the apical impulse may retract away from the palpating finger in systole.
  - Pericardial constriction can be a difficult clinical and echocardiographic diagnosis.
  - It may remain undiagnosed in patients with refractory right heart failure.
- "y" Descent:
  - Prominent "y" descent is a hallmark physical finding of constriction. When present, it is very striking to the trained eye. The neck veins collapse as if a trap door opened. You need to look and listen at the same time. The "y" descent is seen in the neck just after the second heart sound is heard on auscultation. The "y" descent is also out of phase with the palpated carotid impulse (an "x" descent is simultaneous).
  - Pulsed-wave Doppler of hepatic vein flow can be used for confirmation.
  - Doppler examination of the hepatic veins provides the echocardiographic equivalent of the bedside jugular venous inspection.
  - In addition, reversal of hepatic vein blood flow in *expiration* is a useful diagnostic sign. In expiration, the diaphragm stops helping the constricted heart.
  - Transesophageal echocardiography, CT, or MRI may be better suited to evaluate pericardial thickness than transthoracic echocardiography. However,

constriction may be also be caused by stiff pericardium that is not measurably thickened.

- The calcified pericardium "insulates" the heart from intrathoracic respiratory pressure changes and exaggerates respiratory interaction between the ventricles.
- Scanning tip: A septal "bounce" is a respiratory phenomenon that indicates the exaggerated respiratory ventricular interaction of constriction. It may be missed by the interpreter on a short digital loop recording, and should be looked for in real time. A provocative maneuver such as a sniff may be necessary to demonstrate it.
- Biatrial enlargement on echo may be striking (but nonspecific) in constriction. It is due to the chronic elevation in ventricular filling pressures.
- Note: The diagnosis of mild cases of pericardial constriction is usually made in the echo lab, not at the bedside.
- The characteristic bedside examination findings may not be obvious because this is a rare disorder, and clinicians rarely see patients with pericardial constriction.
- However, in *severe* cases of pericardial constriction, the bedside findings may become very obvious. For example, elevated jugular venous pressure may be high enough to manifest itself as persistent jugular venous distention in the *standing* position.
- Sometimes an astute gastroenterologist makes the diagnosis of pericardial constriction by carefully examining the neck veins in a patient referred to GI for ascites.

• Kussmaul sign: *The jugular veins paradoxically expand on inspiration in patients with constriction (normally they collapse on inspiration).*

- Kussmaul sign is characteristic of, but not unique to, constrictive pericarditis. It may be present in patients with asthma, or in patients with right ventricular infarction.
- Furthermore, an exaggerated (hence not paradoxical) drop in systolic blood pressure on inspiration (also described by the astute Kussmaul) is found in cardiac *tamponade* but further confuses, because it can also be present in constriction and is inappropriately called pulsus *paradoxus.*
- Kussmaul had his reasons for picking the "paradoxical" name—the pulse went away, but he kept hearing heart sounds.

Boicourt OW, Nagle RE, Mounsey JP. *The clinical significance of systolic retraction of the apical impulse. Br Heart J.* 1965; 27:379–391.

el-Sherif A, el-Said G. *Jugular, hepatic, and praecordial pulsations in constrictive pericarditis. Br Heart J.* 1971;33:305–312.

Fowler NO, Engel PJ, Settle HP, Shabetai R. *The paradox of the paradoxical pulse. Trans Am Clin Climatol Assoc.* 1979;90: 27–37.

THE LOST ART OF PERCUSSING THE CHEST IN CARDIOMEGALY

"An echocardiographer should never sneer at sending sound into the heart and analyzing the reflected vibrations."

- The art of cardiac percussion is as much tactile as it is auditory.
- A light tap is sufficient. It is not necessary to "percuss to the balcony."
- The total area of dullness to percussion in the normal heart is surprisingly small. Any dullness to percussion of the heart to the right of the sternum suggests cardiac enlargement.
- Percussion of the heart should be performed from the right side of the patient.
- The left hand is placed on the chest when the examiner is right handed.
- The middle finger of the left hand is placed by separating it from the rest of the fingers and hand. It should be placed in the intercostal spaces rather than on top of the ribs. It should be bent in an arc so that only the distal two-thirds of the finger are in contact with the chest wall.
- All soft tissue under the finger should be compressed firmly.
- The fingers of both hands should be as parallel to each other as possible.
- One should strike at a 90-degree angle to prevent sideways displacement of the percussed finger (with resultant muffling of sounds).
- One should strike briskly with motion at the wrist only. The striking finger should be promptly removed to prevent muffling of the elicited percussion sound.
- The point of impact should be just proximal to the nail.

HEPATOJUGULAR REFLUX

- This bedside physical examination sign remains valuable and is easy to do. It is also (more correctly) called the abdominojugular reflux. It is not a reflex.
- It correlates with left atrial pressure and can be performed during echocardiography.
- Transthoracic echocardiography does involve pressure on the abdomen with the transducer to obtain subcostal images.
- Doppler provides real-time changes in flow, and caval inflow can be demonstrated in many patients with Doppler.
- Examination technique:
  - The examiner looks for neck vein distension (with or without pulsation) while firm pressure is exerted over the abdomen in the direction of the spinal column. Fifteen seconds of pressure on the abdomen is adequate for interpretation.
  - The patient has to continue to breathe normally during the time that pressure is being exerted on the abdomen because an unintended Valsalva maneuver will create false-positive neck vein distention.
  - An auscultatory equivalent of a positive hepatojugular reflux also can be sought: The first heart sound may get softer as pressure is being exerted on the abdomen of a patient with heart failure.
- Hemodynamic significance:
  - A positive test is thought to indicate an increased central blood volume. It should also correlate with echocardiographic findings of elevated left atrial pressure.

- Paraphrased from the original description in 1885:
  - An impediment is created to the flow of blood, in either direction, through the inferior vena cava by this maneuver, especially when the liver is enlarged. With each systole an excessive reflux of blood takes place into the superior vena cava. Pulsation, as compared with distension or undulation, is merely one of degree of venous tension.
- Hepatojugular reflux is not specific to any one disorder. It is a consequence of a right ventricle that cannot accommodate augmented venous return.
- Constrictive pericarditis, right ventricular infarction, and restrictive cardiomyopathy are common causes of a positive finding.
- Left ventricular failure also may induce the sign, but only when the pulmonary capillary wedge pressure is >15.
- The one diagnosis *not* seen with hepatojugular reflux is cardiac tamponade.
- It was studied during right-sided cardiac catheterization by measuring changes in right atrial pressure. Bedside observation predicts the response during right-sided cardiac catheterization.
- A positive sign has high sensitivity and specificity for predicting right atrial pressure >9 mm Hg and right ventricular end-diastolic pressure >12 mm Hg.
- In the absence of isolated right ventricular failure, seen in some patients with right ventricular infarction, a positive test suggests a pulmonary artery wedge pressure of ≥15 mm Hg.

Ducas J, Magder S, McGregor M. Validity of the hepatojugular reflux as a clinical test for congestive heart failure. Am J Cardiol 1983;52:1299–1303.

An increase of 3 cm in the height of neck vein distention is a reasonable upper limit of normal.

Ewy GA. The abdominojugular test: technique and hemodynamic correlates. Ann Intern Med. 1988;109:456–460.

A positive test correlates with a pulmonary artery wedge pressure of ≥15 mm Hg.

Sochowski RA, Dubbin JD, Naqvi SZ. Clinical and hemodynamic assessment of the hepatojugular reflux. Am J Cardiol. 1990;66:1002–1006.

Fifteen seconds of pressure are adequate for making the diagnosis.

Wiese J. The abdominojugular reflux sign. Am J Med. 2000;109:59–61.

The sign is absent in patients with tamponade.

VIDEOS

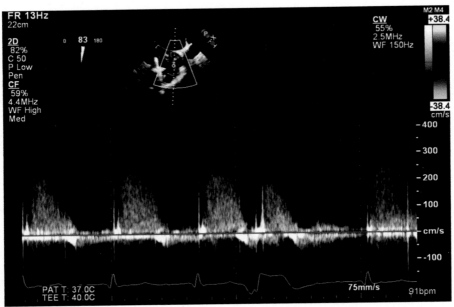

FIGURE 26-3. Tricuspid regurgitation murmurs get louder on inspiration, and softer on expiration, but in this case are apparently not affected by a compensatory pause following a PVC.

VIDEO 26-1. Severe tricuspid regurgitation into the superior and inferior vena cava may correlate with palpable systolic expansion of the liver, and visible prominent systolic expansion of the jugular veins.

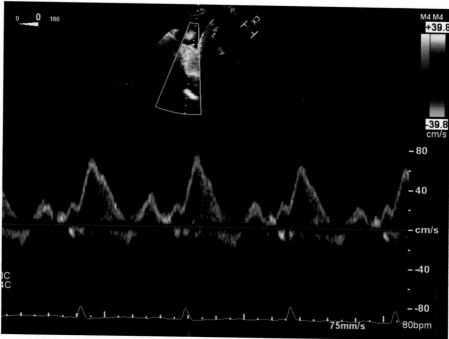

FIGURE 26-4. Pulsed-wave Doppler of SVC flow matches the timing of jugular vein flow on physical examination of the neck.

VIDEO 26-2. Systolic apical excursion of the tricuspid annulus correlates with normal systolic caval inflow in red, and with the normal jugular vein "x" descent on physical examination.

VIDEO 26-3. A pleural rub will disappear during apnea. A pericardial rub will not.

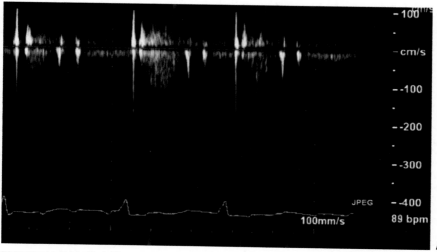

FIGURE 26-5 (A,B). A filter saturation artifact can be used to time the first heart sound. *(continued)*

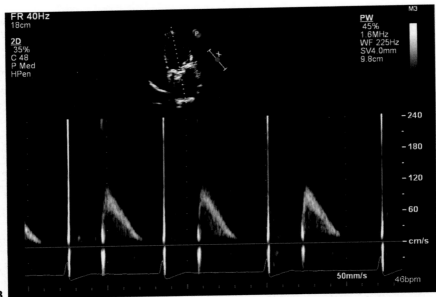

B

FIGURE 26-5 (A,B). *(Continued)* A filter saturation artifact can be used to time the first heart sound.

The Electrocardiogram in the Echo Lab

ECG IN THE ECHO LAB

"Q waves localize myocardial infarction."
"ST segments can diagnose ischemia."

- The 12-lead ECG is a fundamental part of the evaluation for coronary artery disease.
- Scrutinizing the ECG before performing an echo is good patient care.
- Q waves in leads II, III, and AVF help in the sometimes difficult analysis of inferior left ventricular wall motion on the echo.
- Every echocardiographer should be able to recognize classic left ventricular hypertrophy with strain on the ECG.
- Dramatic T wave inversion on the ECG does not always indicate myocardial ischemia. Echo may help.
- An echo with contrast may show a "spade-shaped" left ventricular cavity. This is caused by apical left ventricular hypertrophy. These patients may have giant T wave inversions on the ECG.
- Low QRS voltage on the ECG is important to recognize in a patient with left ventricular hypertrophy on echo. This ECG–echo discordance suggests the presence of an infiltrative cardiomyopathy such as cardiac amyloidosis.
- Patients with Ebstein abnormality of the tricuspid valve have conduction abnormalities on the ECG. Ebstein anomaly is rare, and a suspected diagnosis can be confirmed by echo. It is associated with the more prevalent Wolff-Parkinson-White (WPW) syndrome on the ECG. WPW is more common than Ebstein anomaly. A common phone call from the electrophysiology lab is a request for an echo in a patient with an accessory pathway (WPW).
- Arrhythmias such as atrial fibrillation are sometimes the first manifestation of previously unsuspected valvular regurgitation, cardiomyopathy, and pericardial and congenital heart disorders. Electrophysiologists have many adult patients with congenital heart disease.
- Takotsubo cardiomyopathy may mimic acute anterior myocardial infarction on the ECG.

- If the P wave is >3 mm tall in lead II, look for *right* atrial enlargement on echo.
- If the P wave is prolonged in lead II, and predominantly negative in V1, look for *left* atrial enlargement on echo.
- It is always worthwhile to review the electrocardiogram and to know about disorders that may affect the ECG.

Practical Example

- Causes of tall R waves on the electrocardiogram in lead V1:
  - Posterior extension of inferior myocardial infarction.
  - Right ventricular hypertrophy.
  - Duchenne muscular dystrophy.
  - Dextrocardia.
  - WPW syndrome.
  - Ventricular tachycardia.
  - Normal variant in the young.

Gonzalez-Melchor L, Nava S, Iturralde P, Marquez MF. *The relevance of looking for right bundle branch block in catheter ablation of **Ebstein's** anomaly. J Electrocardiol. 2017;50:894–897.*

Kosuge M, Kimura K. *Electrocardiographic findings of **takotsubo** cardiomyopathy as compared with those of anterior acute myocardial infarction. J Electrocardiol. 2014;47:684–689.*

Murtagh B, Hammill SC, Gertz MA, et al. *Electrocardiographic findings in primary systemic **amyloidosis** and biopsy-proven cardiac involvement. Am J Cardiol. 2005;95:535–537.*

Riera AR, Uchida AH, Schapachnik E, et al. ***Early repolarization** variant: epidemiological aspects, mechanism, and differential diagnosis. Cardiol J. 2008;15:4–16.*

Yamaguchi H, Ishimura T, Nishiyama S, et al. *Hypertrophic nonobstructive cardiomyopathy with giant negative T waves (**apical hypertrophy**): ventriculographic and echocardiographic features in 30 patients. Am J Cardiol. 1979;44:401–412.*

VIDEOS

VIDEO 27-1. Pulmonary vein flow reversal after the P wave in complete heart block.

VIDEO 27-2. Variable degrees of diastolic tricuspid regurgitation in complete heart block.

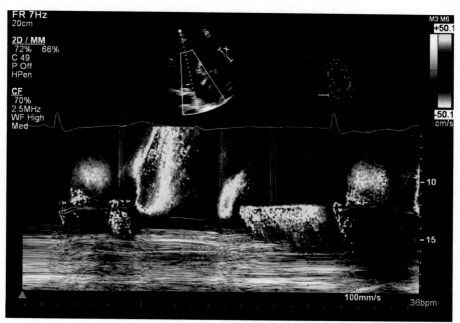

FIGURE 27-1. Diastolic mitral regurgitation in complete heart block.

VIDEO 27-3. Atrioventricular valve motion in complete heart block.

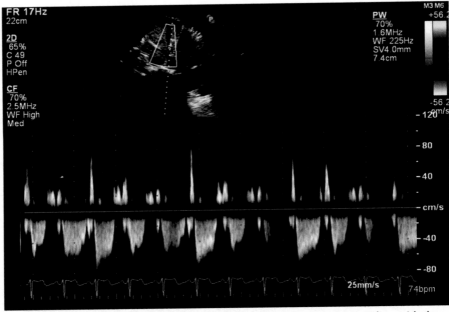

FIGURE 27-2. Hepatic vein velocity spikes (filter saturation artifacts) coinciding with the QRS complexes.

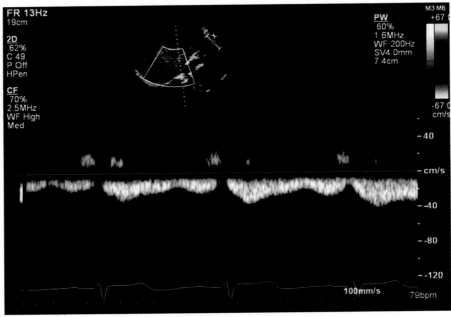

FIGURE 27-3. Hepatic vein flow slowing down at the QRS complex.

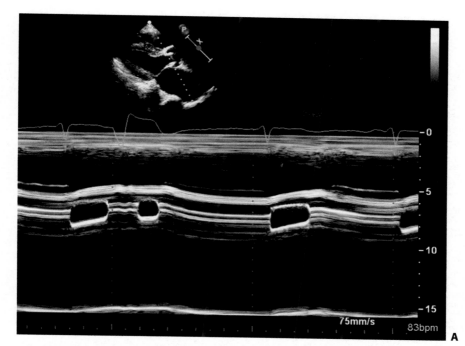

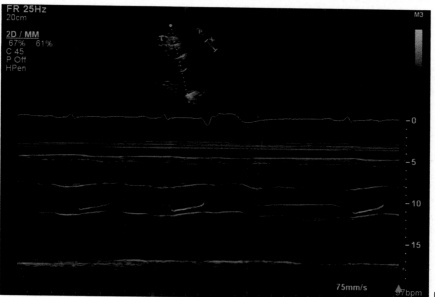

FIGURE 27-4 (A–C). Effect of a PVC on aortic leaflet opening. *(continued)*

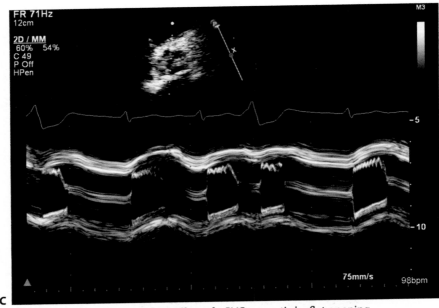

C

FIGURE 27-4 (A–C). *(Continued)* Effect of a PVC on aortic leaflet opening.

VIDEO 27-4. Effect of a PVC on aortic leaflet opening.

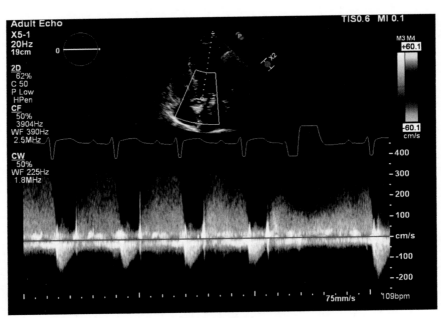

FIGURE 27-5. Effect of a PVC on aortic regurgitation.

VIDEO 27-5. Effect of a PVC on wall motion.

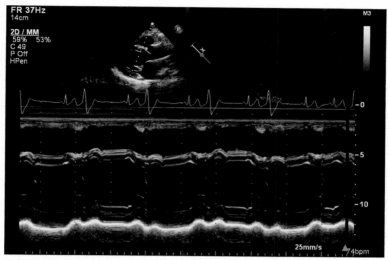

FIGURE 27-6. Bigeminy in dilated cardiomyopathy.

VIDEO 27-6. Variable aortic leaflet opening in atrial fibrillation.

VIDEO 27-7. Wall motion with a PAC.

VIDEO 27-8 (A–C). Wall motion with bundle branch block.

VIDEO 27-9. Left atrial appendage wall oscillations in atrial flutter.

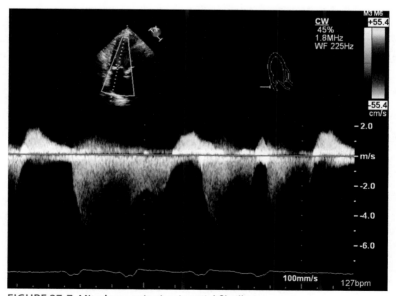

FIGURE 27-7. Mitral regurgitation in atrial fibrillation.

VIDEO 27-10 (A,B). Amyloid cardiomyopathy with low voltage on the 12-lead ECG.

NOTES

CHAPTER 28

Radiology

THE CHEST X-RAY IN THE ECHO LAB

- A phone call may come to the lab asking for an echo because of a finding on a chest x-ray. The following is a very simple but practical guide.
- Lungs: The vascular markings of the lungs may become more prominent. Echo looks for cardiac shunts or causes of left heart failure.
- Cardiac size: The cardiac silhouette may change in size and contour. Echo looks for cardiac chamber size, wall thickness, and function.
- An echocardiographer should be familiar with the rules for normal lung markings on the chest x-ray: The pulmonary vessels branch out in symmetric fashion. They are sharply defined. As they branch out to the periphery, each successive set of branches is slightly smaller—just like in a tree. Normal pulmonary vessels are larger in the *lower* lobes than in the upper lobes.
- Pericardial *calcifications* can be found on the chest x-ray of patients with pericardial constriction. The calcifications may be easier to spot in the lateral films. The calcifications may appear as a hoop, as a band, or as a sheet of calcium.
- Cardiac fluoroscopy can be used to study the function of mechanical prosthetic valves.

X-RAY SIGNS AND EPONYMS

- Vertical heart borders, clear lungs, prominent left pulmonary artery: pulmonic valve stenosis (easily confirmed on echo).
- Pulmonary vessel *pruning* in pulmonary hypertension. There is a sharp decrease in the size of the vascular shadows in the outer regions of the lung fields.
- Rib notching: coarctation of the aorta.
- Waterfall hilum: dilated pulmonary trunk with elevation of the right pulmonary artery due to increased pulmonary flow in a congenital shunt (transposition, tricuspid atresia, truncus arteriosus).
- Shmoo-shaped cardiac silhouette: Left ventricular hypertrophy or enlargement (easy to confirm with echo). The Shmoo was a comic strip creature drawn by cartoonist Al Capp.

- Boot-shaped heart: tetralogy of Fallot—the dilated right ventricle curves around the small left ventricle. The apex of the heart is pushed out and elevated. The cardiac shadow resembles a boot.

Aziz F, Abed M. Coeur en sabot. Cardiovasc J Afr. 2010;21:229–231.

- Right aortic arch: tetralogy of Fallot, or a vascular ring.

Etesami M, Ashwath R, Kanne J, et al. Computed tomography in the evaluation of vascular rings and slings. Insights Imaging. 2014;5:507–521.

- Butterfly or bat wing density of the lung fields: pulmonary edema.

Herrnheiser G, Hinson KF. An anatomical explanation of the formation of butterfly shadows. Thorax. 1954;9:198–210.

- Egg-on-a-string heart: In some patients with transposition of the great vessels, the cardiac shadow resembles an egg that is tilted so that its long axis lies in an oblique position.

Carey LS, Elliott LP. Complete transposition of the great vessels. Roentgenographic findings. Am J Roentgenol Radium Ther Nucl Med. 1964;91:529–543.

- Mogul shadows: The left cardiac border has four bumps (moguls). Enlargement of the *third* mogul happens with left atrial enlargement. First mogul: aorta. Second mogul: pulmonary artery. Fourth mogul: cardiac apex.
- Marked cardiomegaly, expanded right heart border, clear lungs, and small great vessels (small moguls 1 and 2): Look for Ebstein abnormality of the tricuspid valve.

Daves M. Skiagraphing the mediastinal moguls. New Physician. 1970;19:48–54.

- Snowman or figure-of-eight sign: anomalous supracardiac pulmonary vein drainage.

Price EC. Radiologic case presentation. Total anomalous pulmonary venous return to the right superior vena cava. Tex Heart Inst J. 1983;10:93–94.

Snellen HA, Albers FH. The clinical diagnosis of anomalous pulmonary venous drainage. Circulation. 1952;6:801–816.

- Scimitar sign: partial anomalous infracardiac pulmonary vein drainage.

*Brogi E, Bignami E, Sidoti A, et al. Could the use of bedside **lung ultrasound** reduce the number of chest x-rays in the intensive care unit?. Cardiovasc Ultrasound. 2017;15:23.*

*Espinola-Zavaleta N, Játiva-Chávez S, Muñoz-Castellanos L, et al. Clinical and echocardiographic characteristics of **scimitar** syndrome. Rev Esp Cardiol. 2006;59:284–288.*

*Ferrari VA, Reilly MP, Axel L, et al. Images in cardiovascular medicine. **Scimitar** syndrome. Circulation. 1998;98:1583–1584.*

*Gavazzi E, Ravanelli M, Farina D, et al. **Scimitar** syndrome: comprehensive, noninvasive assessment with cardiovascular magnetic resonance imaging. Circulation. 2008;118:e63–e64.*

*Roehm JO Jr, Jue KL, Amplatz K. Radiographic features of the **scimitar** syndrome. Radiology. 1966;86:856–859.*

CHAPTER 29

Internet Resources

GOOGLE SCHOLAR

- The references in the electronic version of this book can be copied and pasted into the Google Scholar search box. *scholar.google.com*
- If the full text is available, it can be saved in your Google Scholar personal library for future reference.
- If access to the full text is restricted on Google Scholar, you can ask your medical librarian for help.
- You can also look for the e-mail address of the corresponding author (usually listed with the free abstract), and ask the author for an electronic copy of the full article.

PUBMED

- U.S. National Library of Medicine (PubMed). *www.ncbi.nlm.nih.gov/pubmed*
- **PubMed** contains more than 30 million citations for biomedical literature from MEDLINE, life science journals, and online books. Some citations include links to full-text content from PubMed Central and publisher websites.
- Search example for pressure half time: *Libanoff Rodbard 1968*
- Many of the guidelines mentioned in this text can be found and downloaded using PubMed.
- **PubMed Central** is a free full-text archive of biomedical and life sciences journal literature at the U.S. National Institutes of Health's National Library of Medicine. *www.ncbi.nlm.nih.gov/pmc*

GOOGLE SCHOLAR VERSUS PUBMED

- Google Scholar is more forgiving during a "copy and paste" literature search compared with PubMed.
- You can copy and paste an entire reference from this book into the Google Scholar search box.

- In PubMed, for best results, you should paste into the search box only *title, journal abbreviation,* and *year* from the references in this book.

Shultz M. Comparing test searches in PubMed and Google Scholar. J Med Libr Assoc. 2007;95:442–445.

GOOGLE IMAGES—SEARCH SUGGESTIONS

- Pictures of prosthetic valves: *Medtronic Hall; Starr Edwards; St. Jude; Carbomedics; Beall; Bjork Shiley strut fatigue.*
- Noonan syndrome: The unique facial features should prompt a search for pulmonic stenosis on echo.
- Holt-Oram syndrome: The "fingerized" thumb should prompt a search for an atrial septal defect on echo.

Böhm M. Holt-Oram syndrome. Circulation. 1998;98:2636–2637.

- "Bread and butter pericarditis" pictures illustrate the surface of the heart in pericarditis. Think about these images when you image the anterior pericardial space from the parasternal window.

Spodick DH. Medical history of the pericardium. The hairy hearts of hoary heroes. Am J Cardiol. 1970;26:447–454.

Homer's Odyssey makes reference to "hairy" pericarditis hearts.

YOUTUBE SEARCH SUGGESTIONS

- *Embryology of the atrial septum* illustrates how a secundum defect is really a defect of the primum septum.
- Search *Paul Wood jugular* to see the neck vein physical exam taught by a master clinician. This helps in the understanding of color Doppler caval inflow patterns.
- *Mantis shrimp* educational videos illustrate the power of cavitation energy.
- Search *Wood units* to see tutorials on vascular resistance.

WIKIPEDIA SEARCH SUGGESTIONS

- Physics terms and units: *wavelength, frequency.*
- Hemodynamic formulas: *Bernoulli, Venturi, Ohm, Laplace, Fick, Poiseuille, Boyle.*
- *Piezoelectric effect.*
- *Electromagnetic spectrum.*
- *Fourier transform.*
- *Radar gun.*

WEBSITES

- Our original 1994 E-chocardiography Journal website: *rwjms1.umdnj.edu/shindler/echo.html*
- Our 2600-member echocardiography group was active from 1998 to 2008. The archive of all the echocardiography discussions is still available. *groups.yahoo.com/group/echocardiography*

- Our 2014 echo textbook: *Practical Bedside Echocardiography Cases.* *www.mhprofessional.com/echoatlas*
- Ask your educational institution to subscribe to Access Cardiology from McGraw-Hill Medical. *accesscardiology.mhmedical.com*

PROFILES OF SELECTED JOURNALS

- A subscription to the printed *Journal of the American Society of Echocardiography* is included in the membership fee for the Society. Guidelines available at *www.onlinejase.com/content/aseguidelines*.
- The *Echocardiography* journal online archive with abstracts (since inception in October 1984) is available at *onlinelibrary.wiley.com*.
- *Cardiovascular Ultrasound* is an open-access journal. There are full-text articles on all aspects of echocardiography, with a particular focus on unusual diagnostic aspects, and expert opinions on new techniques and technologies. They welcome articles with a technical and/or clinical focus and encourage authors to include relevant images, or video files. The authors retain copyright of their work through a Creative Commons attribution license that states how readers can copy, distribute, and use their attributed research, free of charge. *cardiovascularultrasound.biomedcentral.com*
- The *Journal of Diagnostic Medical Sonography* (JDMS) presents the latest diagnostic techniques and interpretation methods, case reports, research applications, and the newest hardware/software technologies and equipment in a variety of specialty areas, including abdominal, breast, echocardiography, neurosonology, Ob/Gyn, and vascular sonography. *journals.sagepub.com/home/jdm*
- The *European Journal of Echocardiography* is published on behalf of the European Association of Echocardiography, a registered branch of the European Society of Cardiology. *www.oxfordjournals.org/our_journals/ejechocard*
  - It publishes articles on the ultrasonic examination of the cardiovascular system, including ischemic heart disease, valve disease, cardiomyopathy, congenital heart disease, and cardiovascular disease.
- *European Heart Journal—Cardiovascular Imaging* is an official publication of the European Association of Cardiovascular Imaging, a branch of the European Society of Cardiology. *academic.oup.com/ehjcimaging/issue*
  - There are articles in all areas of cardiovascular imaging including echocardiography, magnetic resonance, computed tomography, and nuclear and invasive imaging.
- *Circulation* journal contains many landmark cardiology articles. The archive starts in January 1950. *www.ahajournals.org/loi/circ*
- The *Journal of the American College of Cardiology* (JACC) contains many landmark cardiology and echocardiography articles. *www.onlinejacc.org/content/by/year*
- *JACC: Cardiovascular Imaging* publishes research articles on current and future clinical applications of noninvasive and invasive imaging techniques including echocardiography, CT, CMR, nuclear, angiography, and other novel techniques. *imaging.onlinejacc.org*

- *CHEST* is the official publication of the American College of Chest Physicians. There are research articles in the multidisciplinary specialties of chest medicine: pulmonary, critical care, and sleep medicine; thoracic surgery; cardiorespiratory interactions; and related disciplines. There are clinical practice guidelines and consensus statements. Published since 1935. *chestjournal.org*
- *Heart* journal. Formerly the *British Heart Journal*. The archive starts in January 1939. *heart.bmj.com/content/by/year*
- *Texas Heart Institute Journal.* Content beginning in 2014 available electronically only. Content prior to 2014, available at PubMed Central. *thij.org/loi/thij*
- *Open Heart* is an official journal of the British Cardiovascular Society. It is an online-only, open-access cardiology journal dedicated to publishing high-quality, peer-reviewed medical research in all disciplines and therapeutic areas of cardiovascular medicine. *openheart.bmj.com*
  - Opinionated discussions on controversial topics are welcome.
- *The Journal of the Acoustical Society of America.* Archive of article abstracts since 1930. *asa.scitation.org/journal/jas*

Index

NOTES

NOTES

NOTES

NOTES

NOTES

NOTES

NOTES

NOTES

NOTES

NOTES

NOTES

NOTES